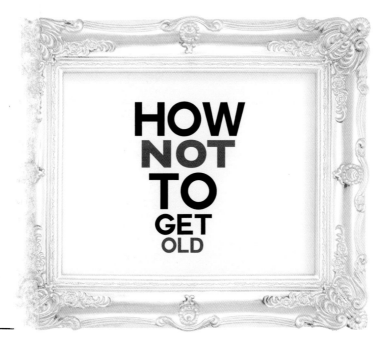

**HOW
NOT
TO**
GET
OLD

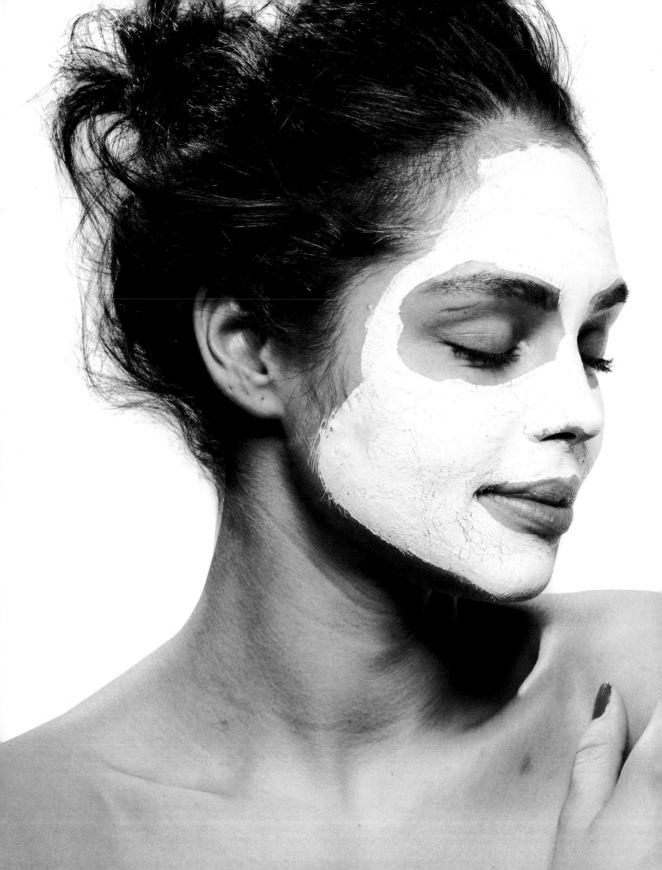

HOW NOT TO GET OLD

YOUR ESSENTIAL GUIDE TO LOOKING AND FEELING YOUNGER FOR LONGER

KAREN DOLBY

BANTAM PRESS

LONDON · TORONTO · SYDNEY · AUCKLAND · JOHANNESBURG

The information in this book has been compiled by way of general guidance in relation to the specific subjects addressed. It is not a substitute and not to be relied on for medical, healthcare, pharmaceutical or other professional advice on specific circumstances and in specific locations. Please consult your GP before changing, stopping or starting any medical or health-related treatment. So far as the author is aware, the information given is correct and up to date as at May 2013. Practice, laws and regulations all change, and the reader should obtain up-to-date professional advice on any such issues. The author and publishers disclaim, as far as the law allows, any liability arising directly or indirectly from the use, or misuse, of the information contained in this book.

Twenty Twenty is one of Britain's foremost producers of award-winning popular television. Its output sells around the globe and spans drama (RTS winner *Garrow's Law*), entertainment (*Styled to Rock*, with Rihanna as Executive Producer) and factual programming (Emmy winner *Brat Camp*, *World's Strictest Parents* and double BAFTA winner *The Choir*).

Karen Dolby has written a wide range of books and was co-author of the best-selling titles *10 Years Younger* and *10 Years Younger Nutrition Bible* published by Transworld. She lives and writes in south London.

TRANSWORLD PUBLISHERS
61–63 Uxbridge Road, London W5 5SA
A Random House Group Company
www.transworldbooks.co.uk

First published in Great Britain
in 2013 by Bantam Press
an imprint of Transworld Publishers

A CIP catalogue record for this book is available from the British Library.

ISBN 978 0 593072 66 0

Addresses for Random House Group Ltd companies outside the UK can be found at: www.randomhouse.co.uk
The Random House Group Ltd Reg. No. 954009

The Random House Group Limited supports the Forest Stewardship Council® (FSC®), the leading international forest-certification organisation. Our books carrying the FSC label are printed on FSC®-certified paper. FSC is the only forest-certification scheme supported by the leading environmental organisations, including Greenpeace. Our paper procurement policy can be found at www.randomhouse.co.uk/environment

Design and art direction: Smith & Gilmour
Photography: Karl Grant
Hair and make-up: Dina Catepole
Stills photography: Fiona Hanson and Anthony Upton
Additional photography: Andrew Lambton (page 6), Paul Farrell (page 30), Wilde Fry (page 124)
Illustration: Johanna Fernihough
Editor: Clare Sayer

Typeset in Gotham and PMN Caecilia
Printed and bound in Great Britain by CPI Group (UK) Ltd, Croydon, CRO 4YY

10 9 8 7 6 5 4 3 2 1

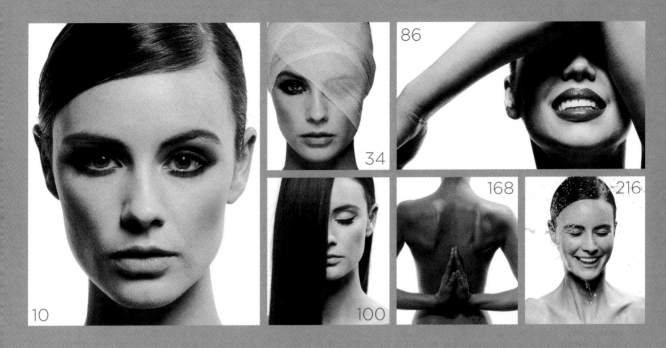

CONTENTS

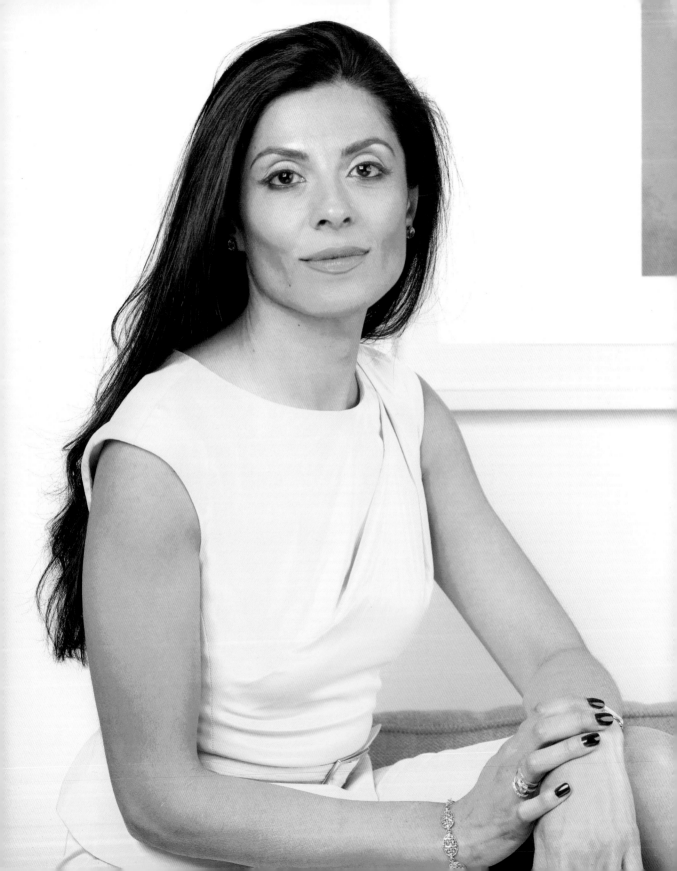

FOREWORD

BY DR ROZINA ALI

Ageing: we're all doing it. It's inevitable and it's gradual. The best any of us can hope for is that it will be as long and slow as possible. But I want more for you.

I think it's perfectly possible to look better as we age: we can mature into our best selves and achieve the face we deserve, not just the one we've earned. My approach to ageing is to embrace the process and aim to age *well* – that is, to be healthy, fit and attractive for as long as you care to be. It takes effort and it takes time. Ageing well is its own process and *How Not to Get Old* is your instruction manual to managing this beautiful change.

Beauty, ageing, appearance – they are all so much more than skin deep. In fact, they go all the way down to the bone. Osteoporotic or thinned bones show more wrinkles; poor diet manifests itself in brittle, pasty skin, thin hair, weak bones and bad teeth; life's worries are etched into frowning faces. But take heart, the converse is also true! Decent diet, regular exercise, healthy lifestyle, sleep, sun protection, skin care and laughter really do work. Essentially, we're performing an intricate dance between extrinsic ageing (the factors we can control) and intrinsic ageing (free radical damage that affects all the body's cells including the skin).

Facial ageing is that infernal trinity of deflation, droopiness and sun-damage. Volume depletion is due to loss of that most-underrated of all tissues – fat. Fat really is the elixir of youth. We don't appreciate it when we have it, we hate it in the wrong places but goodness, do we miss it when it's gone! There are some amazing new research projects under investigation such as autologous fat transfer, whereby your own unwanted fat deposits are harvested and concentrated to replace volume loss in areas such as the face, breasts, or bottom. To me, the future is all about fat.

I THINK IT'S PERFECTLY POSSIBLE TO LOOK BETTER AS WE AGE

Sagging is caused by loss of skin elasticity and structure. Eyes, cheeks, corner of the mouth, jawline, breasts, butt, belly – you name it, all things gradually head downwards. Gravity reigns supreme!

As for environmental damage, look no further than your own personal skin ecosystem of make-up, harsh lotions, sun damage, smoking… you don't need me to tell you that that's never going to end well!

In this book, we show you how to address – and *improve* – specific ageing issues. We use our own trinity of moderation, common truths and new sciences and technologies to delay, derail or even reverse the unnecessary ravages of time. We share with you the judicious use of skin care, modern technologies, non-surgical rejuvenation and surgical methods of combatting ageing.

In my view, well-planned surgery can give you back what you had or better it. Of course, there is no such thing as risk-free surgery. It's a big step that has real risks to go with the rewards. A well-informed patient with realistic expectations is much more likely to achieve an outcome they are happy with and my hope is that *How Not to Get Old* will give you the full, unvarnished truth that will help to inform your decisions. It offers a pragmatic look at all the approaches out there including state-of-the-art science and cutting-edge surgery. Everything that you see has been demonstrated with real, non-airbrushed results on ordinary, honest people.

My interest in this project stems from my knowledge as a scientist and surgeon, as well as my desire to share valuable information. So trust me, I am a doctor and I do know that there really are pills, potions and procedures that work. You just have to know what your problem is, what the treatment does, and how much it can help YOU.

Take your pick of the rich offerings here – and whatever you decide, at least you'll be better informed. And that, dear reader, is the wisdom that also comes with age!

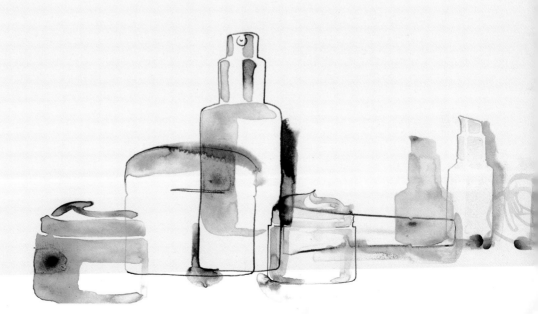

THE
FACE

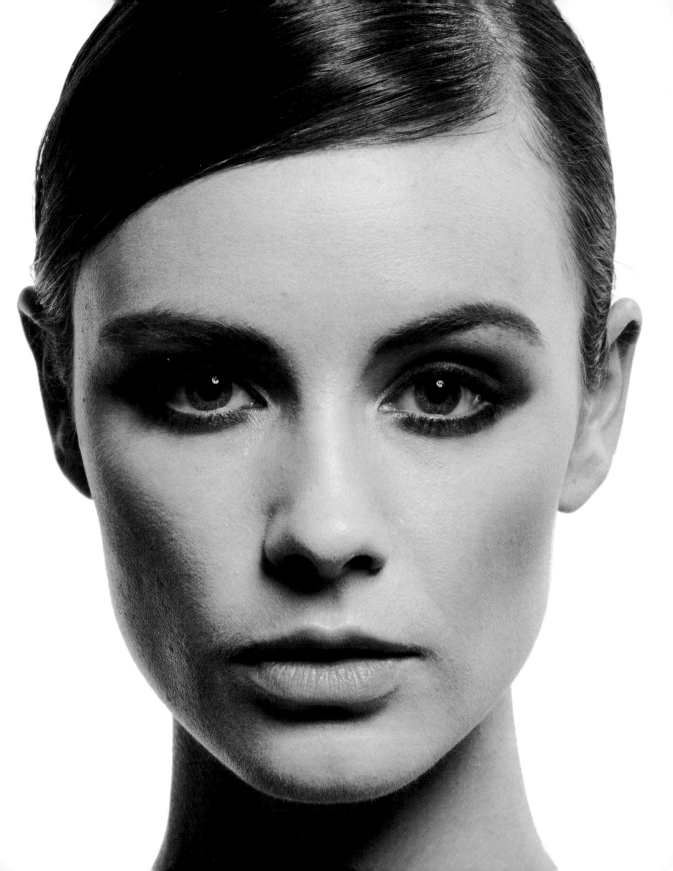

We live in a society where youth is prized. Never before have so many anti-ageing products and procedures been available – open any magazine and you are bombarded with articles and advertisements for the latest youth-enhancing product or treatment. With this comes an increased pressure on everyone to look younger to the point where it can seem no longer acceptable to look your age, let alone old. It's not surprising then that more people than ever are prepared to take drastic measures in an attempt to defy their years. But with so much on offer, it can be hard to know where to start and what really works to enable you to look the best you can, whatever your age.

Nothing gives away your real age quite so obviously as your face. There are other telltale signs, such as your posture, or the inevitable downward pull of gravity on your body, but when deciding someone's age, most people look at the face.

As with most things, prevention is always better than cure and it's never too late to start taking care of your self.

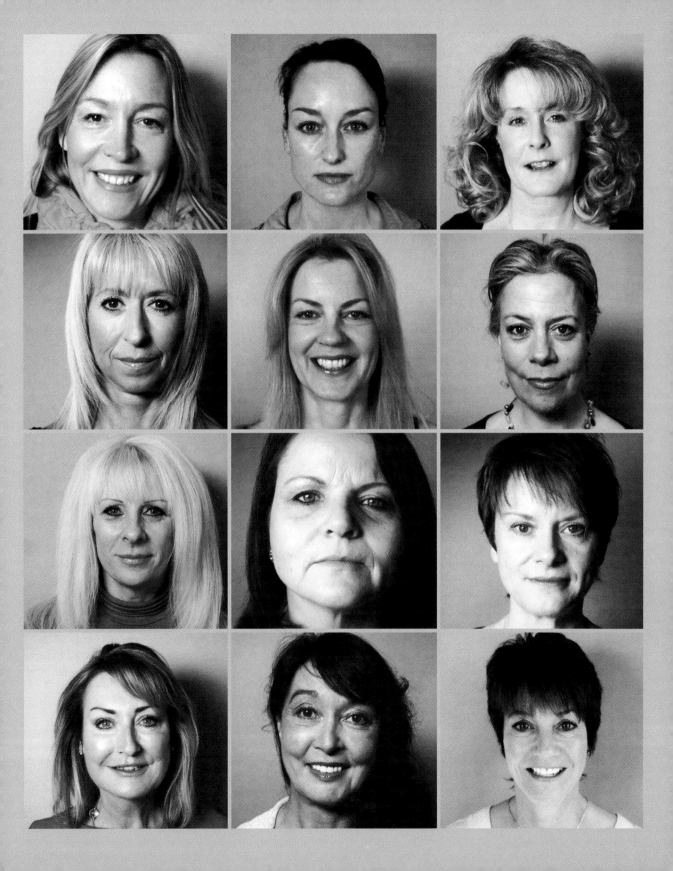

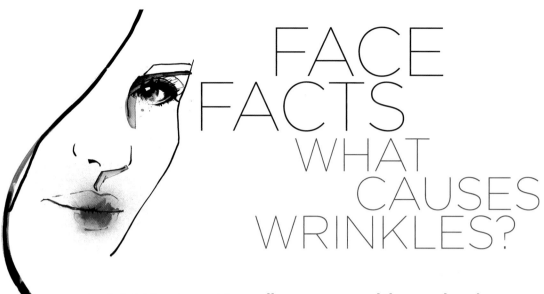

FACE FACTS
WHAT CAUSES WRINKLES?

THE FIRST WRINKLES usually appear around the mouth and eyes. Heredity obviously plays a part but just how well our skin ages is largely down to lifestyle.

THE WORST CULPRIT IS SUN DAMAGE. UVA and UVB rays penetrate the deepest layers of the skin, breaking down the collagen and elastin that are the skin's support structures.

COLLAGEN makes up 70 per cent of skin and is the main structural protein, giving skin strength and maintaining elasticity; without it, skin creases and wrinkles more easily. It's also a vital component of tendons and bones. Elastin is the other main fibrous protein giving skin its bounce. Collagen and elastin are in turn produced by fibroblasts, the most common type of cell in connective tissue. The number and activity of fibroblasts drop as we age.

AS COLLAGEN IS BROKEN DOWN and damaged, the ageing process accelerates. The less collagen we have, the more other factors start to have an impact. Habitual facial expressions etch themselves into lines as the skin loses its ability to bounce back. Frowning may or may not use more muscles than smiling, but furrowed brows lead to deep-set 'elevens' above the bridge of your nose.

NATURAL COLLAGEN AND ELASTIN PRODUCTION also declines with age but there are certain lifestyle factors that can speed up the process.

FREE RADICALS are unstable oxygen molecules that damage cells and slow the production of collagen. They are thought to be a key factor in the ageing process. Sunlight, smoking and air pollution all add to the production of free radicals.

SMOKING can reduce collagen by up to 40 per cent and as it also restricts blood flow to the skin, robbing it of nutrients and oxygen. Wrinkles can start appearing on the faces of smokers as young as twenty. Lines tend to be deeper, skin has a coarser texture and less healthy colour so that by the age of forty, smokers often have as many wrinkles as non-smokers twenty years older than them.

HORMONES also play a part. Reduced levels of oestrogen as we age may decrease collagen levels by 2 per cent a year.

HYALURONIC ACID is a naturally occurring component of skin which helps hydration and elasticity. It also removes toxins, supplies nutrients and supports collagen and elastin. It effectively moisturizes skin from the inside, guarding against wrinkles, but levels fall over time as a result of ageing and the effects of sunlight and pollution.

STRESS, POLLUTION, ALLERGENS, SUNLIGHT AND POOR DIET all cause inflammation which shows itself in the body in stiff, aching joints, irritable bowel syndrome and illnesses such as sinusitis. On the skin, inflammation results in wrinkles and other signs of premature ageing.

EXPERT
ADVICE
HOW TO KEEP YOUR SKIN LOOKING YOUNGER FOR LONGER

Far from being depressing, the message is that what we do makes a real difference and we can all have some control over how well our faces age by following some basic guidelines.

◎ PREVENTION IS ALWAYS BEST What you do in your twenties really affects how well you age in your forties and fifties. Make sure any habits you develop are good ones. But it's never too late to start looking after your skin with a sensible moisturizing, nurturing skincare regime.

◎ WEAR SUNGLASSES with UV protective lenses to avoid developing crow's feet from squinting in the sun. They will also guard against long-term damage to your eyes.

◎ AVOID OVEREXPOSURE TO THE SUN and always wear a sunscreen rated SPF 15 or higher that protects against UVA and UVB. Remember that much of the harm happens by chance whenever we're outside and that tanning is a sign of sun damage. Don't forget your neck, décolletage and the backs of your hands. Nothing ages you faster than sun damage, except smoking…

◎ GIVE UP SMOKING! It's not always easy but this is the one choice you can make that will really affect how old you look. It's estimated that an average smoker ages fourteen years for every ten years of smoking. Do it for your skin, to say nothing of your general health.

◎ SLEEP ON YOUR BACK (this is not a joke). If you always sleep on the same side, the pillow puts pressure on your face leading to lines over the years; lying on your back encourages blood flow and reduces puffiness. Silk pillowcases can also help.

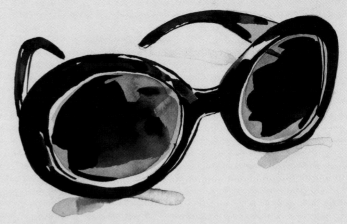

◎ AVOID YO-YO DIETING Constantly losing and gaining weight damages skin. If you need to diet, aim for gradual, sustainable weight loss.

◎ IMPROVE YOUR DIET Balanced nutrition including plenty of fruit and vegetables is essential for healthy skin. B Vitamins biotin and niacinamide (B3) are particularly good for skin, while Vitamins C and E are antioxidant, helping to fight free radicals and protect from sun damage. Vitamin C is also essential for collagen production while Vitamin A helps to repair and maintain skin tissue.

◎ DRINK PLENTY OF WATER to keep skin hydrated and plump out fine lines. This is such a simple tip, but it really makes a visible difference to your skin.

◎ EXERCISE It goes without saying that exercise, fresh air and a good night's sleep all work wonders for your looks.

DID YOU KNOW?

SUN DAMAGE
ACCOUNTS FOR UP TO 90 PER CENT OF WRINKLES AND OTHER SIGNS OF PREMATURE AGEING.

SUN WARNING

◎ LONG-SPECTRUM UVA rays penetrate cloud and mist.

◎ THE SUN'S RAYS are at their strongest between May and October, and between 10am and 3pm. Reflection from water, snow, sand and even concrete magnifies their effect.

◎ AT HIGH ALTITUDES the atmosphere is thinner, allowing more harmful ultraviolet radiation (UVR) to reach us. UVR levels rise by 4–5 per cent for every 1,000 feet of altitude.

◎ UVA RAYS PENETRATE more deeply into the skin than UVB ones, reaching the dermis, the living layer of skin.

◎ FAR FROM PROTECTING your skin, a tan is the skin's response to cellular DNA damage.

◎ SUNBURN AND SKIN CANCER were believed by experts to be caused by UVB, while UVA was responsible for photoaging. The reality is more complex and both contribute to ageing and the risk of skin cancer.

◎ CHEMICAL SUNSCREENS should be applied around twenty minutes before sun exposure so that your skin has time to absorb them.

◎ MINERAL SUNSCREENS work immediately because they form a physical barrier on the skin surface.

◎ AS A GENERAL GUIDE, if your skin normally burns after twenty minutes in the sun, an SPF 15 sunscreen will protect you for fifteen times longer. But damage can be invisible, so dermatologists recommend reapplying cream after two hours.

◎ OLDER SKIN benefits from the addition of liposomes or essential fatty acids to rehydrate skin and enable the sunscreen to retain its effectiveness for longer.

A WORD OF WARNING
Always check with a doctor or dermatologist, especially if you notice any changes in pigmentation or moles.

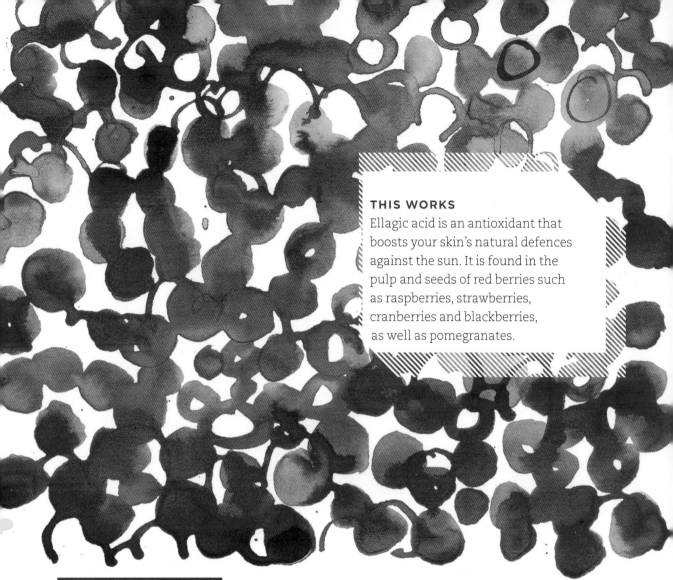

THIS WORKS
Ellagic acid is an antioxidant that boosts your skin's natural defences against the sun. It is found in the pulp and seeds of red berries such as raspberries, strawberries, cranberries and blackberries, as well as pomegranates.

DID YOU KNOW?
IT'S NOT ALL BAD. WHO DOESN'T FEEL AND LOOK HAPPIER WHEN THE SUN'S SHINING? AND PROVIDED YOU PROTECT YOUR SKIN ADEQUATELY, IT'S ALSO GOOD FOR YOU, HELPING TO FORM ESSENTIAL VITAMIN D WHICH IS VITAL FOR HEALTHY, STRONG BONES.

THE DIFFERENCE BETWEEN MEN AND WOMEN

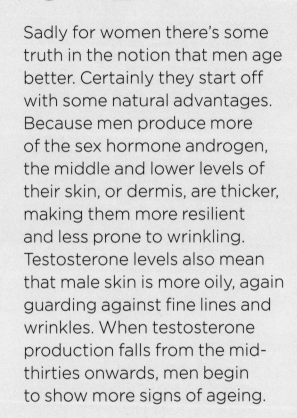

Sadly for women there's some truth in the notion that men age better. Certainly they start off with some natural advantages. Because men produce more of the sex hormone androgen, the middle and lower levels of their skin, or dermis, are thicker, making them more resilient and less prone to wrinkling. Testosterone levels also mean that male skin is more oily, again guarding against fine lines and wrinkles. When testosterone production falls from the mid-thirties onwards, men begin to show more signs of ageing.

SMOKE WARNING

It's estimated that for every minute you spend smoking, you lose a minute of your life. Smoking ages the skin, heart, lungs and can trigger early menopause, cancer and osteoporosis, cutting life expectancy by around ten years.

SMOKING AGES SKIN by triggering the production of an enzyme that breaks down collagen, attacking skin's elasticity. Smokers who sunbathe age even faster as UV rays accelerate this reaction.

TOBACCO SMOKE RESTRICTS BLOOD FLOW to the skin and deprives it of nutrients.

IT PARTICULARLY ROBS THE SKIN of vitamin C's antioxidant protection and vitamin A's moisturizing defence.

SKIN IS LEFT DRYER, GREYER and with a noticeably more coarse texture. Stress lines develop around the mouth and eyes.

SMOKERS OFTEN DEVELOP HOLLOW CHEEKS from the action of drawing on a cigarette as well as the telltale puckering around the lips.

However…just two weeks after giving up you should notice a marked improvement in the way your skin looks as circulation improves and nicotine and carbon monoxide levels fall.

SOUND SKINCARE

The starting point for anyone wanting to look younger for longer has to be a good skincare regime. This is for the long term – not a quick fix but a sound investment for your future and has to be followed rigorously every day. Don't worry – it doesn't have to be elaborate or take hours. Just a few simple steps make all the difference.

◎ IT'S IMPORTANT TO ALWAYS cleanse your face. In the morning this freshens and prepares your skin for any other products you use. You're aiming to clean skin without sapping the moisture, so look for hydrating cleansers rather than soap. Cleansers such as E45 or aqueous cream are cheap but effective.

◎ ALWAYS FOLLOW CLEANSING with a moisturizer, preferably one with anti-ageing ingredients. Moisturizer reinforces the skin's naturally protective, oily surface layer, the stratum corneum, which can quickly become dehydrated, dry, flaky and wrinkly.

◎ DON'T FORGET SUN PROTECTION You may prefer to combine this with your moisturizer or other face cream but if you are on holiday somewhere sunny or during the summer months when rays are at their strongest, it is often more effective to use a separate sunscreen with SPF 15 or higher.

◎ MOISTURIZER not only locks in hydration and moisture, it also protects skin from the environment and the harmful effects of free radicals. It soothes and calms any irritation and forms a good base for other cosmetics and make-up, helping them last longer and look better.

◎ AT NIGHT THE ROUTINE should be repeated to remove any dirt that's accumulated during the day, and to allow your skin to breathe and repair itself – vital for youthful-looking skin. You may prefer to use a different moisturizer at night, particularly targeted at anti-ageing, with extra antioxidants.

◎ SKIN AROUND THE EYES is more delicate and should be treated differently. Use a specific eye make-up remover (although some people swear by Johnson's Baby Oil or Vaseline). Follow with an eye cream that reduces puffiness and works on fine lines.

◎ FROM TIME TO TIME it is worth adding extra, targeted products to keep your skin healthy. Seasonal changes such as dryness in winter or uneven pigmentation at the end of summer, periods of stress and changes in your hormone levels can all wreak havoc with your complexion.

◎ TRY TO EXFOLIATE once a week to remove dead skin. This helps to keep your complexion glowing and youthful. There are many good exfoliating creams, washes, masks and peels to choose from, or you can achieve the same result with a clean, warm flannel. Squeeze out excess water and gently massage your face using a circular motion. Take care not to pull the skin and finish by lightly pressing the warm cloth against your face. Moisturizing masks work particularly well after exfoliation. Face scrubs, particularly those containing high levels of fruit acids, proteolytic enzymes and glycolic acid, help strip away the dull, lifeless surface layers of the skin. It is vital that you moisturize and protect the soft, new skin that emerges.

THIS WORKS
Aqueous cream, which costs less than £4 for a sizeable pot, is a non-greasy cleanser and moisturizer that leaves a layer of oil on the skin surface that prevents moisture evaporating.

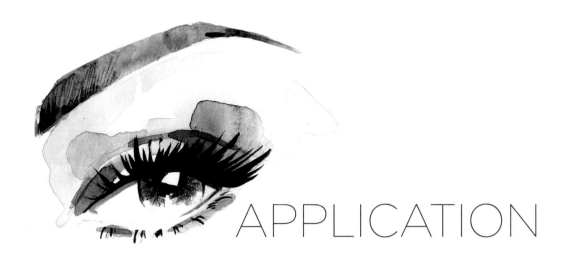

APPLICATION

The way you apply products also makes a difference. Always be gentle, using light circular movements to cleanse or moisturize. It can be helpful to warm creams in the palm of your hand before application.

FOR EYE CREAM less is definitely more. Take a tiny amount, roughly the size of a grain of rice, and warm between your two little fingers. Pat it lightly into the skin below your eyes and across the brow and socket line until it is absorbed.

EXPERT TIP
Eye cream also works effectively on the lips. Any eye cream left on your fingers can be patted into the skin around your lips and your nasolabial lines running from your nose to your mouth.

WHAT TO LOOK FOR IN AN ANTI-AGEING CREAM

While scientists may not have found the age-defying miracle cure just yet, research has revealed a number of key ingredients that slow down and may even reverse some of the signs of ageing. It is worth looking out for these when choosing an effective skin cream.

◉ **VITAMIN A** comes in a few forms including retinoids, tretinoin and retinol, which vary in their degree of intensity. Tretinoin can only be prescribed by a doctor and was originally used to treat acne but it was noticed that a side effect was that patients looked younger. It boosts collagen production, thereby plumping skin and reducing the appearance of fine lines, sun damage and discolouration. This is quite a harsh ingredient and the skin has to build up tolerance to it. Typically, products contain no more than 0.3 per cent and should be applied at night only as it is unstable in sunlight. For anti-ageing, dermatologists would usually recommend its use just twice a week as it is very drying, so skin should also be well moisturized. Pure retinoids are also only available only through prescription, while retinol, a milder form of vitamin A, can be used in cosmetics.

A WORD OF WARNING
Prescription-strength Vitamin A should not be used when pregnant, when trying to get pregnant or when breastfeeding.

◎ **VITAMIN C** is an antioxidant that helps to protect skin from free radical damage. It is also vital for the production of collagen and it seems that it is important not just to eat it but also to include it in our skin cream. However, you need a high concentration for it to make any impact and as Vitamin C can become oxidized if exposed to the sun, there are only a few stable forms which have been developed for topical use. Most are water-soluble and therefore unable to penetrate the skin's epidermis, but **tetrahexyldecyl ascorbate** is more lipid-soluble which means it is more effective.

◎ **VITAMIN B3 OR NIACINAMIDE** improves the skin's moisture barrier which helps the natural production of collagen. It also strengthens the surface layer of the epidermis, the stratum corneum. It can even help to reverse the signs of past damage by encouraging skin renewal and improving the appearance of uneven pigmentation and enlarged pores.

◎ **HYALURONIC ACID** is a naturally occurring component of connective tissue in the body, giving flexibility to blood vessels and cartilage as well as the skin. It also boosts the skin's moisture and hydration levels, giving it a youthful, healthy appearance. Unfortunately, hyaluronic acid levels decline with age adding to the development of fine lines and wrinkles. Cosmetic-grade hyaluronic acid can help reverse the decline and stimulate the skin's own production.

◎ **PEPTIDES** are short chains of amino acids (tiny fragments of protein molecules) that occur naturally in the skin. They are the building blocks for the natural production of the proteins collagen and elastin. Hailed as a Botox effect in a cream, peptides are a growing trend in anti-ageing skincare and can improve hydration in the stratum corneum (the surface layer of the epidermis) by boosting collagen levels which decline with age, thereby plumping the skin and giving it elasticity. **Oligopeptide-34** is one type of peptide which has been clinically proven to reduce wrinkles and fine lines. When tested, it also proved to be the most effective skin whitener not derived from hydroquinone, which is restricted in many countries. Various other peptide ingredients have been developed such as **Matrixyl**, **RonaCare Cyclopeptide-5** and **Pal-KT** and laboratories are working to produce longer-chain peptides and better results.

◎ **ALPHA HYDROXY ACID (AHA)** was one of the first products found to have anti-ageing properties. AHAs are derived from foods, for example: glycolic acid from cane sugar, lactic acid from sour milk, malic acid from apples, citric acid from citrus fruits and tartaric acid from wine grapes.

◎ **AHAS EXFOLIATE** by helping skin shed the unhealthy dead outer layers which can build up, allowing other moisturizers and treatments to penetrate the skin and work more effectively. They are particularly useful for treating sun-damaged skin which has thickened and become rough and uneven in tone, and for smoothing surface lines. Both skin tone and texture improve after exfoliation.

◎ **FOR ANY TOPICAL TREATMENT** to be effective, it must penetrate the outer layer or epidermis to reach the living dermis. Glycolic acid has the smallest molecular size of all the alpha hydroxy acids and so has the best chance of being absorbed. Glycolic and lactic acids are also the most researched forms of AHAs.

◎ **BETA HYDROXY ACID (BHA)** is similar to AHA but is only available as salicylic acid. It is used in lower concentrations than AHAs but, for both, the pH of the product should be between three and four in order to effectively exfoliate skin. If the pH is lower than three it will be too irritating for most skin types.

◎ **EPIDERMAL GROWTH FACTORS (EGF)** are the newest buzzwords in the cosmetics industry. They are a group of cells with a number of specialized functions, most importantly, the activation of cellular proliferation and differentiation. Basically, they turn essential cellular activities on and off, playing a role in increasing cell production and division, as well as the production of blood vessels, collagen and elastin.

EGFs are present in the platelet-rich plasma (PRP) treatment used in Dr Sister's so-called 'Dracula Therapy' (see page 60). There is some controversy around the use of EGFs at the moment, as many dermatologists believe the molecules are too big to penetrate the epidermis. Cosmeceutical brands such as Medik8 advise their use with a dermaroller to ensure the product penetrates through to the dermis.

◎ **LIGHTENING AGENTS** are used to treat hyperpigmentation as a result of sun damage. A number of agents are known to be effective including hydroquinone, kojic acid, arbutin and azelaic acid, all of which work by inhibiting melanin production. In Europe, hydroquinone can only be prescribed by a doctor as it can be harmful.

WHAT TO LOOK FOR IN A SUNSCREEN

No guide to anti-ageing creams would be complete without mention of sunscreens, which are the best defence against early ageing. Most skincare experts would recommend regular use as their number one anti-ageing tip.

PROVING THAT A SKIN CREAM REALLY WORKS AS AN ANTI-AGEING TREATMENT CAN BE A DOUBLE-EDGED SWORD FOR COSMETICS COMPANIES. IF A PRODUCT IS CATEGORICALLY SHOWN TO BE EFFECTIVE, IT HAS TO BE LICENSED AS A MEDICINE, MAKING IT AVAILABLE ON PRESCRIPTION ONLY – MADNESS IN MARKETING TERMS. CONSEQUENTLY MANY ANTI-AGEING CREAMS AVAILABLE ON THE HIGH STREET REMAIN ON THE SURFACE AND DON'T PENETRATE THE SKIN.

◎ **AVOBENZONE** is a chemical screen that offers good protection against UVA but not UVB rays.

◎ **OCTOCRYLENE AND OXYBENZONE** are chemical screens that are effective against UVB rays.

◎ **TITANIUM DIOXIDE OR ZINC OXIDE** are physical, mineral sunscreens that are effective across the UVA and UVB spectrum – micronized versions mean they no longer leave that unattractive white residue on the skin.

◎ **MEXORYL SX** is one of a new generation of organic filters that is UVA protecting.

◎ **ANTHELIOSSX** combines **MEXORYL SX** with **avobenzone** and **octocrylene** to give effective broad-spectrum sun protection.

◎ **RESEARCH SUGGESTS** that the inclusion of antioxidants, particularly **Vitamins C and E**, can help prevent cell damage by reducing the free radicals and inflammation caused by sun exposure, guarding against wrinkles, photopigmentation or sun spots, and even skin cancer.

THIS WORKS
Laboratory studies carried out by Ian Hamley, Professor of Chemistry at Reading University, found that when concentrations of the pentapeptide Matrixyl 3000 were high enough they significantly boosted the production of collagen. The question now is how much is needed to make a difference.

THE COST OF YOUTH
Matrixyl can be found in:
◎ Olay's Regenerist Daily 3 Point Treatment Cream – £15.32 for 50 ml
◎ L'Oreal Collagen Filler – £10.99 for 30 ml
◎ St Ives Collagen Elastin Facial Moisturizer – £8.44 for 30 ml
◎ Skin Doctors Cosmeceuticals 2600 Retanew – Retinol Wrinkle Reduction – £25.56 for 50 ml
◎ Tranquillity Skincare Youth Re-Surge Anti Wrinkle Cream – £30 for 30 ml
(Source: Daily Mail, 6.3.2013)

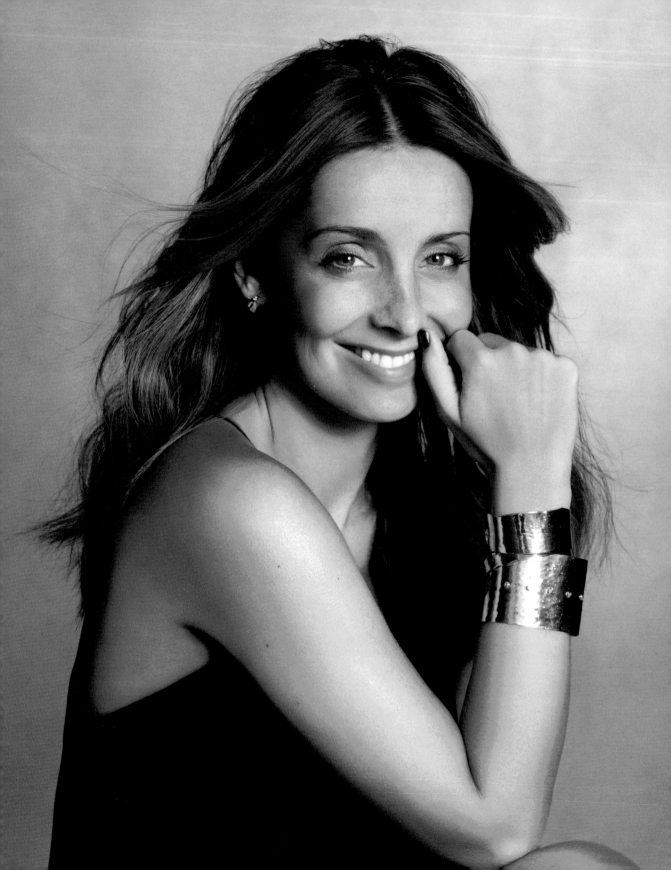

AGEING NATURALLY
LOUISE REDKNAPP

Presenter, businesswoman, fashion lover, former member of nineties R&B girl band Eternal, successful solo singer, awarded *FHM*'s sexiest woman of the year 2004, famously married to Liverpool and England footballer Jamie Redknapp and mother of two boys – even Louise Redknapp thinks ageing can be tough for women. 'There's just so much pressure to stay looking young, and there are so many different products on the market.'

Louise firmly believes that what you put into your body has a direct impact on the way you look and that a balanced diet and exercise can all help to maintain a healthy, youthful appearance.

During the series *How Not to Get Old*, she looks at some of the more preventative measures people can take to hold back the years. 'I think alternative routes to anti-ageing have a real place and I'm keen to champion natural treatments,' she explained.

And Louise has put into practice what she believes. Last year she launched a make-up range with her friend and make-up artist Kim Jacobs. Called 'Wild About Beauty', the range is paraben-free and uses natural extracts and oils including rosewater, argan oil, beeswax, sea marine extract and green caviar for their anti-ageing, anti-inflammatory qualities, as well as their ability to soothe, moisturize and hydrate skin.

She views make-up as a great tool for making you feel good about yourself, giving you confidence and a sense of youth. 'Yes to some degree it's an illusion, but it helps you make the best of yourself – much like a well-cut dress or great pair of jeans. A spring in your step can take years off your age.'

LOUISE'S TOP TEN BEAUTY TIPS

1 SKINCARE As we get older our skin naturally loses some of its luminescence. To try and combat this I use products that act specifically on boosting radiance, such as Wild About Beauty's Rose Water Illuminating Serum. This product is packed with violet light-reflecting particles that really help to bring back brightness and luminosity. Just a few drops on to the skin, on its own or under foundation, gives your complexion an instant lift.

2 SKINCARE REGIME Whatever your age, looking after your skin should be a priority. Fresh, clear skin is the single thing that will give you confidence. If your skin looks tired and dull, you're never going to feel great. As you get older, use products that are more moisturizing to recreate the dewy-skinned look of youth. I use Dr Francis Prenna Jones Formula 2006 morning and night. This is a simple to use, all-in-one miracle worker that cleanses, tones and moisturizes and tackles pigmentation. My main tip would be to not overcomplicate your skincare regime; the simpler it is the more likely you are to stick to it!

3 FOUNDATION If ever I am asked for just one beauty tip I always stand by my rule of 'less is more'. Though as we get older this can become harder to stick to. Skin tends to get drier and we start to notice the somewhat inevitable signs of ageing. In an attempt to hide these 'imperfections' we are often tempted to wear more make-up.

In fact, a heavy foundation is likely to make the skin even drier and therefore accentuate any fine lines, wrinkles and age spots. A hydrating, tinted moisturizer is often the best choice to give you more radiant, youthful-looking skin. A moisturizing skin primer can also provide a good base for other products but avoid powder, which tends make any lines more obvious rather than disguising them. If you're concerned about shine, go for a mattifying balm rather than a powder. Keeping skin protected is equally important so ensuring your face make-up has an SPF is crucial.

4 SUN DAMAGE It's not only dangerous for your health but also incredibly ageing. Wild About Beauty Sheer Glow Moisture Tint covers all bases perfectly – it leaves skin hydrated with a dewy, natural-looking finish and the SPF 20 ensures you are always protected in the sun.

HOW
NOT
TO
GET
OLD
32
**AGEING
NATURALLY**

5 BROWS As we age our brows often thin out. Don't be tempted to over pluck or draw in eyebrows using a harsh pencil as this gives a 'hard' look that can be very ageing. A thicker, softly defined eyebrow helps frame the face and give an overall more youthful look. I love the Laura Mercier Eyebrow Pencil in soft brunette. It is the ideal colour for me and has a really soft texture – both these aspects are so important for natural-looking brows.

6 LIPSTICK The older we get, the harder it is to wear dark, matte lipsticks as they can feather into the lines on our lips and are often too severe against ageing skin. Sheer, lighter and more emollient formulas will look softer and more youthful. To further eliminate feathering, try using a lip pencil but always make sure this colour isn't too contrasting to the colour of the lipstick as this can create a harsh look and add years to you. Wild About Beauty's double-ended Lip Pencil Duos offer a lipstick in a lovely lightweight formula and have a perfectly matched lip liner.

7 EYES AND LIPS Never do too much eye and lip together in one look. Far from making you look younger, it'll add on ten years. If you want a heavier eye, then compensate by using a sheer, tinted lip balm. Generally it's better to avoid hard lines and keep colours sheer and simple.

8 EXERCISE I find that keeping myself fit through exercise is a foolproof way for looking and feeling younger. I favour Pilates as it makes my body feel stronger and leaner than any other form of exercise. Try to find an exercise that you can enjoy. It will not only improve your appearance but also your general health and mental well-being.

9 NUTRITION Certain foods can really help. My mum swears by fish oils and I try to eat oily fish at least twice a week. Almonds are packed with protein and essential fatty acids – they make the ideal snack. Avocados are also full of essential fatty acids, minerals, protein and antioxidant vitamins, including Vitamin E which helps to iron out wrinkles, and are great for glossy hair. Summer fruits are the perfect excuse for juicing – delicious, good for you and an easy way to your five a day. I'm also a big fan of ginger. It really wakes up your whole body combined with lemon juice in hot water.

10 SLEEP A lack of sleep ages from the inside out, leaving us looking pale and tired with dark under-eye circles. Therefore, if we want to look and feel youthful, it is crucial to get sufficient sleep. People find various remedies and routines to help facilitate a good night's rest, from a relaxing bath before bed to herbal medicine or reflexology. Try experimenting until you find something that works best for you. Personally, I find reflexology is really effective at relaxing the body and mind and normally a peaceful night's sleep follows.

TREATMENTS FOR THE FACE

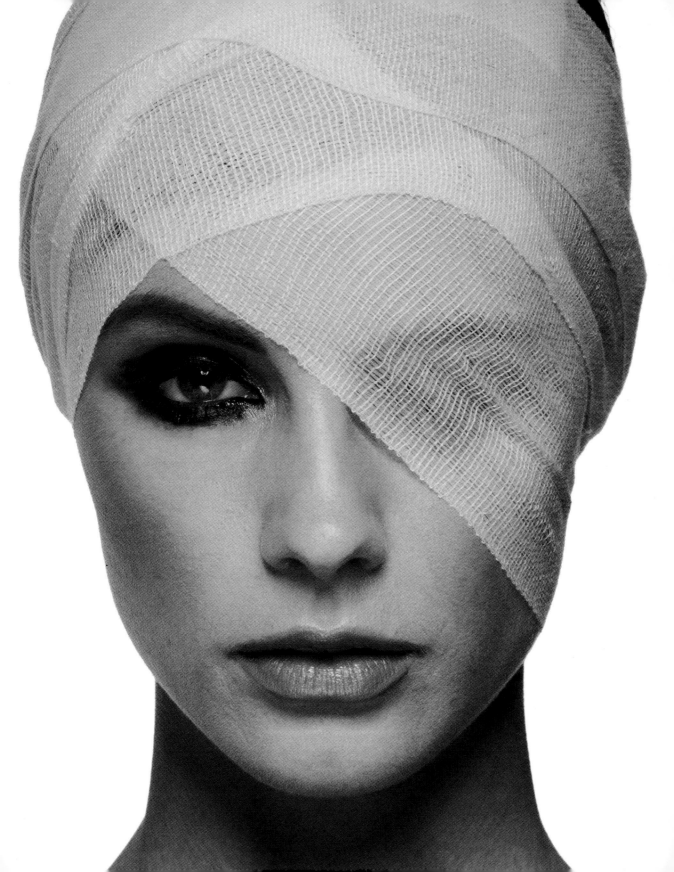

There are times when we want a cure, no matter how good our care and prevention has been. We cannot stop all signs of ageing, and neither should we want to. Lines show our expressions and reflect our character, but sometimes we need a little extra help to look healthy, glowing and rejuvenated.

The range of treatments available has never been broader – from facials to facelifts the quest for youth means the anti-ageing industry is booming. The claims are impressive but can you believe the hype? Understanding what's available and what you can reasonably expect from a procedure helps when it comes to deciding what options are right for you.

ANTI-AGEING TREATMENTS
FACIALS AND MASSAGE

There are a number of anti-ageing facials on offer, designed to tone and firm the face and brighten the complexion. These tend to be aimed at prevention and maintenance and won't necessarily have much impact on deep lines. A good facial or massage should, however, improve the health and strength of your skin, leaving it naturally glowing and radiant.

When choosing a facial, look for one that offers something different from what you can achieve by yourself at home. A powerful, deep massage or a treatment using a machine or equipment will deliver products on a cellular level to penetrate into the skin.

The professional strength products used in these treatments, including peels, vitamins and peptides, should also be more effective than those you can buy for yourself. They will target the skin surface as well as the lower layers of the epidermis and dermis, stimulating fibroblast and collagen production, and all the natural processes of renewal that gradually slow with age.

When opting for any treatment, it's always worth doing your research. At the simplest level, some therapists massage better than others and achieve more impressive results.

TREATMENTS
FOR THE
FACE

ACUPRESSURE OR FACIAL REFLEXOLOGY

Essentially this is acupuncture without the use of needles – pressure is applied to the same pressure points. It helps relieve stress and tension, which can show on the face as wrinkling and premature ageing. Acupressure also improves circulation and lymphatic drainage, stimulating nerves and tissue, rejuvenating the face and leaving you feeling energized. It has an instant soothing effect on the skin and has been described as 'unfreezing your face, relaxing it into a glowing, unfraught, chilled-out version of its former self'. Like all reflexology it aims to improve general well-being, working on physical, hormonal and emotional imbalances that can affect the skin's health and appearance.

AROMATHERAPY MASSAGE

The essential oils used have a direct effect on mood while the massage relaxes muscles and improves circulation. Oils such as rosehip can be particularly rejuvenating for ageing skin.

FACIAL ACUPUNCTURE

The therapist starts by taking a detailed medical history after which very fine disposable needles are inserted into specific pressure points to create a 'micro-trauma'. This encourages increased blood flow and nutrients to remove toxic waste and energy blockages, stimulating collagen and elastin and kick-starting the skin's natural rejuvenation process. Your face often reflects your mood and internal state; worry lines form on the brow while laughter lines tend to point upwards.

As this is a holistic treatment, needles are also placed around the body. After 30–45 minutes, the needles are removed and the face is massaged with an oil mixed to suit individual needs.

A course of treatments is usually recommended but you can see results after just one session. Fans of facial acupuncture report a noticeable lift with facial tension lines far less obvious, wrinkles smoother and skin generally plumper. It is needles without the Botox® but just as effective – plus your mind feels calmer and your body is energized.

COST: FROM £50 A SESSION, DEPENDING ON THE PRACTITIONER.

HOW
NOT
TO
GET
OLD
38
**TREATMENTS
FOR THE
FACE**

OXYGEN FACIALS

A machine directs pure oxygen at the skin and is used in conjunction with anti-ageing serums, antioxidants and hyaluronic acid to plump skin and improve elasticity.

COST: FROM £60.

CACI (COMPUTER AIDED COSMETOLOGY)

A micro-electric current is passed through the facial muscles to exercise and tone. Initially three treatments a week are needed for four weeks, with further follow-up sessions every six to eight weeks.

COST: FROM £50 PER SESSION, ALTHOUGH PRICES CAN VARY WIDELY DEPENDING ON THE PRACTITIONER AND TREATMENT.

GENTLE SKIN PEEL

A light peel containing alpha hydroxy acid (AHA) or glycolic acid can help reduce the appearance of fine lines around the eyes or mouth as well as brighten dull skin. It removes a layer of dead skin cells, boosting your complexion and improving the texture. Results usually last between three and six months.

COST: FROM £70.

THIS WORKS

For an instant fix for tired-looking skin, give yourself a face massage. While you are cleansing, gently but firmly massage along the cheekbones, jawline, forehead, brow and temples. Finish by hanging your head upside down for a moment to encourage blood flow to your face.

Lightly massaging on either side of the bridge of your nose with your middle fingers will help to reduce fluid retention and puffiness around the eyes, especially first thing in the morning.

HOW
NOT
TO
GET
OLD
39
TREATMENTS
FOR THE
FACE

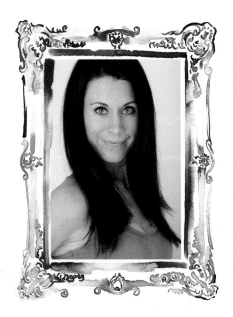

EXPERT PROFILE
DANIELLE COLLINS, FACE YOGA

In her quest for natural anti-ageing treatments, Louise Redknapp visited face yoga expert Danielle Collins at her private studio in Bath for a group class.

Danielle Collins believes that most people want to look naturally good for their age. Through her Face Yoga programme she offers a holistic, long-lasting anti-ageing alternative to surgery and Botox®, working with the mind and body as well as the face. A session gives you time to yourself – to think, unwind and relax. You leave feeling positive and rejuvenated.

She has been teaching her method for over eight years after students at her body yoga classes asked for exercises specifically designed for the face. She initially became interested in yoga and nutrition after successfully treating her own ME (chronic fatigue syndrome).

THE METHOD

Danielle created a twenty-minute programme to be practised daily, six days a week. Her Face Yoga programme uses traditional techniques dating back thousands of years to give safe, natural anti-ageing results. According to Danielle visible benefits include reduced lines and wrinkles and skin that is lifted and firm, with improved tone. Other outcomes include a reduction in headaches and eyestrain and the relaxing of tension, giving an energetic appearance to the face and a healthy glow. Face Yoga also gives a holistic feeling of well-being.

HOW
NOT
TO
GET
OLD
40
TREATMENTS
FOR THE
FACE

THE FIVE ASPECTS TO FACE YOGA

★ **Face exercise** Just as your body needs regular exercise to stay toned and firm, the fifty-seven muscles in the face and neck also need to be exercised. As they become stronger through exercise they are lifted and firmed and the skin attached to the muscles is also lifted and tautened, thereby reducing lines and wrinkles. As the muscles are much smaller than those in the body, it takes a lot less time for them to increase in strength and tone.

★ **Face massage** By regularly massaging the face using the techniques from Danielle's Yoga Method, you will increase blood circulation and lymph flow and remove toxins. This will reduce poor skin tone, puffiness and dark circles and allow the skin to look healthier and more youthful. The massage techniques will also increase the amounts of the natural plumping agents collagen and elastin, which will mean a firmer and healthier complexion.

★ **Acupressure** This age-old technique works by pressing on certain points on the face, increasing the flow of the subtle energy or *prana* in the face. This therefore reduces tension, increases circulation and gives a healthy glow to the skin.

★ **Relaxation** Learning to relax tension in the face will help to reduce and prevent the deep-set lines and wrinkles caused by stress, squinting or grimacing. Face Yoga allows you to relax the face correctly, giving it a more open, youthful look.

★ **Well-being** The well-being aspect of the Danielle Collins Face Yoga Method will also do wonders for your overall health and happiness. Taking time to relax, doing something for you, and knowing you will look and feel better as a result may mean you also notice yourself feeling calmer and more energized, as well as looking younger and healthier. What happens on the inside radiates on the outside.

HOW
NOT
TO
GET
OLD
41
TREATMENTS
FOR THE
FACE

Altogether there are eighteen face yoga exercises which take twenty minutes to complete. These are the three most popular

★ The 'V': to reduce lines and wrinkles around the eyes and to make the eyes more open and energized

Put both your middle fingers together between your eyebrows then apply pressure to the outer corners of your eyes with your index fingers. Look up and start to move the lower eyelids upwards, making a strong squint. Relax and repeat six more times. To finish, squeeze your eyes shut for ten seconds then relax.

★ The Smile Smoother: to reduce lines around the mouth and to lift and firm the cheeks and jaw

Hide your teeth with your lips and make an 'O' shape with your mouth. Then smile as wide as you can, while keeping the teeth hidden. Repeat six times. Next, hold the smile shape and place one index finger on the chin. Then start to move your jaw up and down as you tilt your head back. Relax and repeat twice more.

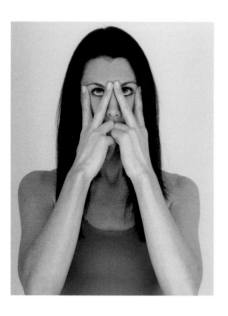

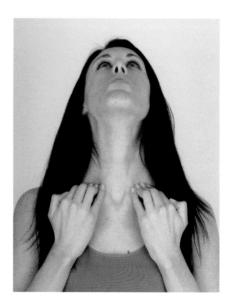

HOW
NOT
TO
GET
OLD
42
TREATMENTS
FOR THE
FACE

★ The Giraffe: to tone and lift the neck area

Looking straight ahead, place your fingertips on the top of your neck and pull the skin down as you tilt your head back. Bring your head back down and repeat twice more. Then jut your lower lip out as far as possible, place your fingers on your collarbone and point your chin upwards, pulling the corners of your mouth down. Hold for four deep breaths.

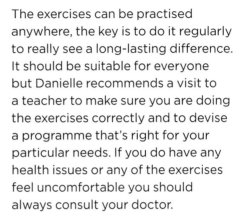

The exercises can be practised anywhere, the key is to do it regularly to really see a long-lasting difference. It should be suitable for everyone but Danielle recommends a visit to a teacher to make sure you are doing the exercises correctly and to devise a programme that's right for your particular needs. If you do have any health issues or any of the exercises feel uncomfortable you should always consult your doctor.

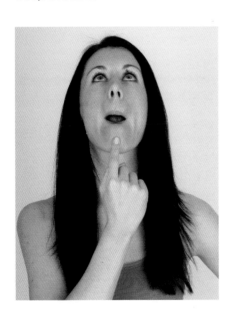

HOW
NOT
TO
GET
OLD
43
TREATMENTS
FOR THE
FACE

FROM HOLLYWOOD TO THE HIGH STREET

In the quest for effective anti-ageing facials, practitioners are turning to increasingly bizarre ingredients to get results. Often originating in LA, with high-profile endorsements, they quickly catch on elsewhere.

PLACENTA SERUM

The Lancer Clinic in Beverly Hills is the pioneer of this treatment, which uses placenta extracts from New Zealand sheep – the only ones considered pure enough. Nutrient-rich stem cells are harvested from amniotic cells (so no animals are harmed) and then mixed with gold flakes before being massaged into the skin. Victoria Beckham and Simon Cowell are said to be fans of this facial, which prompts the production of collagen and brightens the skin.

COST: £320 FOR THE FACIAL AND £70 FOR 35ML OF GOLD STEM CELL SERUM.

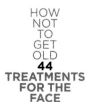
HOW
NOT
TO
GET
OLD
44
**TREATMENTS
FOR THE
FACE**

SNAIL MUCUS

Snail mucin extract is a complex blend of proteins, glycolic acids and elastin, renowned for its regenerative properties – restoring damaged tissue and replenishing moisture in skin. It is also an effective treatment for acne and scarring. If large African snails trailing their way across your face is not your idea of a relaxing facial, Katie Holmes is said to be a fan of Dr Jart+ Premium Time Returning Serum, which contains 77 per cent snail mucus. Another option is Masqueology Cell Renewal Masque With Snail Secretion Filtrate.

COST: DR JART+ PREMIUM TIME RETURNING SERUM $54; MASQUEOLOGY CELL RENEWAL MASQUE $24, BOTH AVAILABLE FROM SEPHORA IN THE US.

THE GEISHA OR BIRD POO FACIAL

Nightingale droppings have been used by Japanese geishas for centuries as an effective skin cleanser. Containing the amino acid guanine and nitrogen-rich urea, the facial was developed by Shizuka Bernstein in New York. The sterilized droppings are powdered and mixed with rice bran, which exfoliates and reduces pores, and water, before being spread on the skin. An antioxidant-rich green tea mask finishes the treatment to leave the skin bright, smooth and supple with fine lines eased. Both Victoria and David Beckham are reported to be fans.

COST: ABOUT £135.

SNAKE SERUM

A cream rather than a facial. The neuropeptide Syn-ake is a synthetic version of the poison from the temple viper, a venomous snake indigenous to Malaysia. It is used in face creams to stun the skin into remaining tight, decreasing the appearance of wrinkles. Described as a non-surgical alternative to Botox®, it has several celebrity fans.

COST: ABOUT £100, DEPENDING ON THE BRAND.

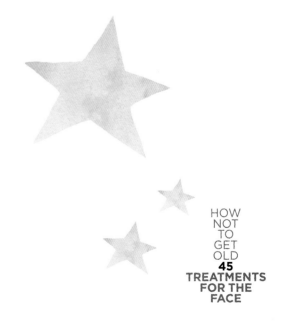

HOW
NOT
TO
GET
OLD
45
TREATMENTS
FOR THE
FACE

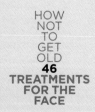

CLINICAL TREATMENTS

Anti-ageing procedures for men and women have never been more popular with the numbers of face, brow and neck lifts, and eyelid surgery increasing. Figures for Botox, fillers and fat transfers are also rising.

Rajiv Grover, a consultant surgeon and president of the British Association of Aesthetic Plastic Surgeons (BAAPS) said, 'The growth rates for surgical facelifting and other anti-ageing procedures showed a double-digit rise, despite a double-dip recession.'

HOW
NOT
TO
GET
OLD
46
**TREATMENTS
FOR THE
FACE**

TRENDS AND FIGURES

◎ BAAPS' 230 SURGEONS carried out 43,172 surgical procedures in 2012, a slight increase on the previous year.

◎ BREAST AUGMENTATION was the most popular at 9,843 procedures, although that represented a slight fall on the previous year. This was probably due to concerns over the dangers of PIP breast implants rupturing and leaking non-medical grade silicone into the body.

◎ OPERATIONS ON MOOBS fell 18 per cent from 2011 with 642 men opting for surgery. There was speculation this was because more men were heading to the gym, possibly inspired by the 2012 Olympics.

◎ THE SAME REASON may account for the 10 per cent fall in liposuction and tummy tucks.

◎ ANTI-AGEING SURGERY was generally on the rise. The number of facelifts increased by 14 per cent, brow lifts by 17 per cent, and eyelid surgery by 13 per cent.

◎ FAT TRANSFERS – taking fat from one part of the body and injecting it into another, invariably the face – also rose by 13 per cent.

HOW
NOT
TO
GET
OLD
47
**TREATMENTS
FOR THE
FACE**

BUYER
BEWARE!

◎ THE COSMETIC SURGERY industry in the UK is now worth in the region of £900 million each year. It's estimated that up to five million people would seriously consider some form of cosmetic surgery and many procedures, particularly for fillers and Botox, are routinely on offer on the high street. But there is growing concern about the lack of regulation and the fact that people may unwittingly be placing themselves at risk.

◎ ALMOST HALF THE CLAIMS for cosmetic surgery that has gone wrong are successful, compared with 30 per cent for general medical compensation. There has been a significant rise in claims over the last five years with legal action for breast surgery, facelifts, eyelid operations, nose reductions and weight loss procedures accounting for 80 per cent. A range of blunders have left patients with asymmetrical features, scarred, burned, or with health problems including breathing difficulties. Individual payouts of up to £500,000 reflect the seriousness of the claims.

◎ SURGEONS THEMSELVES are calling for official regulation of the industry. Dr Clare Gerada, chair of the Royal College of General Practitioners said, 'The use of cosmetic surgery has ballooned over the last few years. It is important that whilst surgery is deceptively easy to obtain, standards of care are always upheld, and that profit should never take precedent over high-quality care.'

◎ IT IS HOPED that the government review led by Sir Bruce Keogh will result in enforceable legislation. 'We're handing the government the scalpel. It's time to cut out bad practice,' says BAAPS president Rajiv Grover.

HOW
NOT
TO
GET
OLD
48
TREATMENTS
FOR THE
FACE

IS YOUR SURGEON QUALIFIED?

◎ MOST IMPORTANTLY you want to be sure that your surgeon is properly trained and qualified. Even non-surgical procedures can have serious side effects and you want to know you are going to get the best care and limit any risks as far as possible.

◎ IN THE UK, all surgeons who have six years training in plastic surgery, in addition to their general medical training, are listed on the General Medical Council's (GMC) specialist plastic surgery register. This is separate from the specialist register. You can obtain a copy from the GMC, 350 Euston Road, London NW1 3JN or from its website at www.gmc-uk.org.

◎ THE BRITISH ASSOCIATION of Plastic Surgery (BAPS) is part of the Royal College of Surgeons and has 225 members, all on the GMC register, and all qualified to carry out cosmetic surgery, although many concentrate on regenerative or other plastic surgery rather than cosmetic procedures. You can contact BAPS through its website at www.baps.co.uk.

◎ MEMBERS OF BAPS who specialize in cosmetic surgery are further registered with the British Association of Aesthetic Plastic Surgeons (BAAPS). There are 140 BAAPS surgeons at present, all of whom are recognized by the NHS as experts in their field and fully qualified to carry out procedures including breast, facial or laser surgery, facial fillers and Botox®. The letters FRCS and PLAS after a surgeon's name show that he or she is a member of the RCS and specialist plastic surgeons. You can find further information on BAAPS website at www.baaps.org.uk.

◎ BOTH BAPS AND BAAPS will give you advice about surgeons and procedures.

HOW
NOT
TO
GET
OLD
49
**TREATMENTS
FOR THE
FACE**

WHAT TO LOOK FOR WHEN CHOOSING A COSMETIC SURGEON

◎ YOUR STARTING POINT should always be your GP who can refer you to a registered plastic surgeon and give you general medical advice. Your own GP will also be able to pass on any relevant medical information to your surgeon, which may affect your treatment or recovery.

◎ THOROUGHLY CHECK a potential surgeon's qualifications and area of expertise. Find out how many operations or procedures like yours they carry out each year and ask to see photographs of the results.

◎ BE FULLY INFORMED about the procedure you are considering. In particular find out what the risks and limitations are, and remember that no surgery or procedure is totally risk-free.

◎ YOU SHOULD ALWAYS see your surgeon before an operation. Counsellors or sales people are not qualified to discuss your surgery or advise on whether it is right for you. And they are certainly not medical experts.

◎ MAKE SURE you have all the details, including the results you can expect, possible side effects, how long it will take and the recovery period, including post-op precautions.

◎ BE CERTAIN that this is the right treatment for you, considering your age and lifestyle. It is also best to avoid surgery if you have recently experienced a major life change or emotional upheaval.

◎ NEVER LET YOURSELF be pressurized into going for surgery and always try to get unbiased information. It is a serious commitment and you should feel completely happy about your decision.

HOW
NOT
TO
GET
OLD
50
**TREATMENTS
FOR THE
FACE**

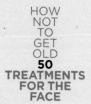

◎ BAAPS SURGEONS typically spend thirty minutes to an hour just on the initial patient consultation.

◎ PERSONAL RECOMMENDATION is ideal. If you know someone who has had the same procedure and are impressed with the results, ask where they had it done and who was the surgeon.

◎ BE CAUTIOUS of any clinic offering free consultations or special deals and avoid booking fees or non-refundable deposits. You should be free to change your mind at any point.

◎ BAAPS ALSO WARNS against travelling long distances for surgery as this could cause problems with follow-up checks or if there are complications. Be especially careful before considering cosmetic surgery tourism. Financially it may seem like a good deal but a significant number of people need further treatment when they return home, either from surgical complications, because they have been discharged too soon, or because they are just not happy with the result.

BAAPS recommends that you make sure you feel completely comfortable with your choice of surgeon and clinic. It warns, 'Many practitioners may boast impressive sounding qualifications but these can have little meaning. Organizations associated with and preferably based in the Royal College of Surgeons will demonstrate acceptable standards of practice, i.e. those which you can reasonably expect of surgeons and doctors in general. Hospitals which have strong links with NHS consultants and practice will also adhere to these standards and so offer some level of reassurance. The BAAPS can help you find a properly credentialed surgeon in your area.'

HOW
NOT
TO
GET
OLD
51
**TREATMENTS
FOR THE
FACE**

DERMAL FILLERS

A large number of different fillers are available which can be injected into outpatients. They are used to ease wrinkles, firm facial contours and replump cheeks and lips; results can last for up to a year.

Fillers can be broadly divided into biocompatible and synthetic. Biocompatible fillers are safer and resorbable – meaning they can be broken down and assimilated back into the body. Synthetic fillers are permanent but are rarely recommended by experts as there are so many risks associated with them, including rejection, the formation of hard lumps and slippage or movement. In addition, if there is a bad reaction, removal is almost impossible. Biocompatible fillers include:

COLLAGEN These were the first fillers to appear on the market but because the solution is prepared from human and bovine sources there can be problems with severe allergic reactions. A pre-test is needed before injecting a bovine preparation because of the high risk of sensitivity. The results are also very short-lived and so this type is now rarely used.

AUTOLOGOUS CELL THERAPY Skin cells are processed into a collagen suspension for injection. Two or three treatments take place over a period of three months. This is a costly treatment and there is some debate about how effective it is, although advocates claim it gives better, longer-lasting results.

POLYATIC ACID (SCULPTRA®)
This works to stimulate the body's own fibroblast and collagen production. It can be used on all parts of the face, neck and décolletage. It can also add volume to hollow or baggy areas such as rings under the eyes or folds around the chin and is used to treat scars. Two sessions at least fifteen days apart are usually sufficient; Sculptra works over time with the full effect taking four to six weeks to develop, and improvements lasting one to two years. It should always be injected by a qualified, specially trained practitioner as fibrous nodules can appear if it is wrongly injected.

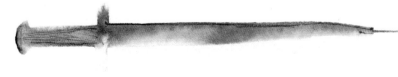

HOW
NOT
TO
GET
OLD
52
**TREATMENTS
FOR THE
FACE**

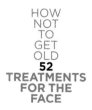

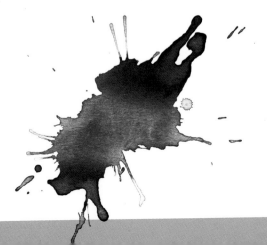

HYALURONIC ACID (RESTYLANE AND JUVEDERM) There are various types of hyaluronic filler suitable for different areas including cheeks, lips and around the mouth and eyes. An experienced practitioner will advise on which would work best for you. A gel is injected which acts like a cushion and boosts the skin's hydration, plumping and smoothing wrinkles and folds. Results are instantaneous and usually last between six and nine months, sometimes up to a year. Maintenance treatments are then needed. Because hyaluronic acid is natural in origin, you do not need an allergy test but there is a very small (1 per cent) risk of an adverse reaction, including granular inflammation.

COST OF FILLERS: FROM £100, ALTHOUGH THIS VARIES ACCORDING TO THE FILLER USED AND THE AREA BEING TREATED.

DID YOU KNOW?
BAAPS surgeons regularly turn away one in five potential patients. The main reasons why are:
◎ The procedure is unsuitable or unnecessary, e.g. too young for a facelift.
◎ The patient has unrealistic expectations about surgery, e.g. wanting to look like a particular celebrity.
◎ There are medical reasons why surgery would be dangerous, including obesity, a heart condition or being a smoker.
◎ BAAPS president Rajiv Grover concludes, 'In the right circumstances, aesthetic plastic surgery can have a positive impact on a person's life. Under the wrong conditions – particularly in a sales-driven, "stack em high" environment – the results can be no less than catastrophic.'

HOW
NOT
TO
GET
OLD
53
TREATMENTS
FOR THE
FACE

A WORD
ON DERMAL FILLERS

In 2012, more than two-thirds of BAAPS surgeons saw patients with complications caused by temporary dermal fillers (including hyaluronic acid), and nearly half saw problems with semi- or permanent fillers (for example Bio-Alcamid and Aquamid). Some of these were so serious they required surgery to correct the damage caused, but an alarming number were considered untreatable.

Synthetic fillers are particularly problematic and BAAPS does not recommend their use. There have been problems including infection, severe allergic reactions and slippage leading to deformity. PMMA, a type of semi-permanent filler used in the cosmetic industry, is made from the same product used in the manufacture of plastic windows.

Mr Niall Kirkpatrick is a craniofacial surgeon, whose day job involves working with cancer patients. He is also the country's expert on removing dermal fillers that have gone wrong from patient's faces. Sometimes the dermal fillers cause necrosis, where the cells die, and skin blackens or collapses in on itself.

Unlike Botox®, a regulated drug that is also used for medical purposes, dermal fillers are classed as 'medical devices', putting them in the same category as plasters or disposable gloves. In the EU fillers are barely regulated, meaning that there are over 160 different types on the market. This is in sharp contrast to the US, where fillers *are* regulated and only six different types are considered safe to be sold. This also means that absolutely anyone can inject dermal fillers – at present you could set up your own clinic today if you

HOW
NOT
TO
GET
OLD
54
**TREATMENTS
FOR THE
FACE**

wanted – without any training at all – and that's exactly what many people do. Key figures from within the aesthetics industry have been calling for urgent changes to the current situation.

They have received a big boost in their efforts from Bruce Keogh's long-awaited Review into the cosmetics industry which was made public on 24 April 2013. Commissioned by the government following the PIP breast implant scandal, the main recommendations are for better regulation, better training and proper means of redress if things go wrong. The intention is to create a freely available, thriving industry but, crucially, one that is safe and properly regulated.

Bruce Keogh admitted that he was surprised at the lack of regulation for non-surgical treatments, saying, 'A person having a non-surgical cosmetic intervention has no more protection and redress than someone buying a ballpoint pen or toothbrush.' He was particularly concerned about the pressure consumers come under to sign up immediately, and with misleading buy-one-get-one free-type offers where you cannot be sure of quality.

Dermal fillers were seen as a crisis waiting to happen. To combat the problem the main recommendations are:

◎ All dermal fillers should be prescription only.
◎ Every practitioner should be properly qualified, from cosmetic surgeons to those offering injectables, and they should have the skills and expertise to perform procedures safely and to a high standard.
◎ Appointment of an ombudsman to oversee all private health care, including cosmetic procedures.

Consultant Plastic Surgeon and BAAPS President Rajiv Grover commented on the report, 'We are thoroughly relieved that the Review has come to the same conclusions as we have over the years, specifically the urgent need for dermal fillers to require a prescription for use. This measure will kill three birds with one stone: regulating which ones come onto the market, who can inject them and automatically banning their advertising.'

HOW
NOT
TO
GET
OLD
55
**TREATMENTS
FOR THE
FACE**

THE Y-LIFT

Also known as the 'lunchtime facelift' or 'Thirty-minute facelift'. The process actually takes 30–45 minutes, results are immediate and patients can return to most normal activities afterwards. Improvements last up to two years. It claims to be a facelift without the knife, restoring features and facial structure to a younger appearance. It's so-called because the facial contours can be seen as a Y and as we age the arms of the Y widen and sag.

The Y-Lift was pioneered by Dr Yan Trokel in New York and uses a specialized titanium instrument which is inserted beneath the skin and manoeuvred to lift and contour the muscles, fat and skin. Hyaluronic acid is then used to hold the newly lifted position and the titanium tube is removed. The face is then sculpted to accentuate and make the best of the patient's features. There are no incisions or stitches and no general anaesthetic is necessary.

As well as accentuating cheekbones and the under-eye area, it can also be used to lift the brow, reshape the chin and jawbone and to lift and revitalize the skin.

COST: FROM £2,500.

DERMAROLLER

Also known as micro-medical skin needling, the Dermaroller has been described as looking like a mini medieval instrument of torture. Skin is numbed first, then the device is rollered across the face to make thousands of microscopic needle holes in the dermis, increasing blood flow, prompting skin to produce collagen and generate new cells. It is used to treat signs of ageing, sun damage, wrinkles, acne scars and stretch marks. For a few days, skin looks almost sunburned and needs extra care, especially moisturizing. It is often most effective on the lower part of the face; skin will appear generally plumper, smoother and firmer but results are not instant. Three sessions carried out six weeks apart are usually recommended with visible results after the second session. Be careful as there are imitations around and treatment should always be by a trained medical practitioner or authorized clinic. There is a risk of infection from the puncture wounds.

COST: ABOUT £250 PER SESSION.

THIS WORKS
Studies have shown that trauma to the skin through tiny puncture wounds (like those made by machines like the Dermaroller) can dramatically increase natural collagen levels.

HOW
NOT
TO
GET
OLD
56
**TREATMENTS
FOR THE
FACE**

FAT TRANSFER OR LIPOFILLING (SOMETIMES REFERRED TO AS A FAT GRAFT FACELIFT)

This procedure takes fat from elsewhere in the body to volumize and rejuvenate the face. The fat is usually taken from one or more small incisions in the abdomen or thigh, or as part of a liposuction procedure.

The fat cells are then centrifuged and filtered before being injected back into cheeks, temples, chin, the lips or under the eyes to plump and preserve facial contours. It may be that stem cells are introduced back into the face along with the fat cells to stimulate fibroblast and collagen production, but further research is needed to know for sure. The fact that the patient's own tissue is used helps to avoid allergic reactions.

Minute amounts of liquid are evenly distributed so that the injected fat is surrounded by healthy tissue. Local anaesthetic is applied first. The procedure takes about an hour and there will be bruising, swelling and some tenderness afterwards.

The use of icepacks is recommended and the swelling tends to be worse on the third day, after which it gradually goes down. It usually takes about a week to ten days to feel confident about going out and the remaining bruises can be covered with make-up. There will be an initial check-up after five to seven days and a follow-up appointment three weeks later.

Up to 30 per cent of the fat cells don't survive and there is a further resorption of between 20 and 50 per cent. The final result is achieved after three months, after which a second session may be thought necessary.

Risks include infection and asymmetry but results can be impressive, correcting deep wrinkles and folds and improving skin quality, as well as adding volume to the face. The effects last up to six months.

COST: ABOUT £2,500, DEPENDING ON THE PRACTITIONER.

HOW
NOT
TO
GET
OLD
57
**TREATMENTS
FOR THE
FACE**

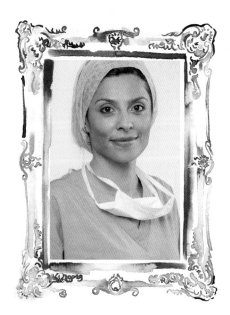

EXPERT PROFILE
DR ROZINA ALI

How Not To Get Old's plastic surgery expert Dr Rozina Ali is a highly skilled breast and micro-vascular reconstruction plastic surgeon. She is also an expertly trained cosmetic surgeon with a wealth of experience in procedures including facelifts, upper and lower eyelid surgery, tummy tucks and liposuction, as well as a range of specialist non-surgical rejuvenation techniques, including HA fillers, Botox®, lipofilling (fat injections), transdermal mesotherapy, Pellevé radiofrequency skin tightening and therapeutic or active skincare.

I try to understand what people really want and work with them to get the best results... Being comfortable in your own skin is the ultimate luxury.

She firmly believes that nothing is as good as nature and the best anti-ageing strategy is to look after yourself. She sees skincare as an integral part of grooming – the equivalent of visiting the hairdresser, the gym or the dentist for regular care and maintenance.

Like many of the best cosmetic surgeons, she is of the 'little and often' school when it comes to procedures like Botox and fillers. After all, you don't hesitate before treating a headache or toothache – why wait if there's a solution available to fix the perceived problem. Used sensibly, she thinks rejuvenation treatments can help people look their best and feel confident. They can remain relevant well into theirs seventies, eighties and beyond. 'I don't call it "anti-ageing", I just call it making the most of yourself.'

HOW
NOT
TO
GET
OLD
58
**TREATMENTS
FOR THE
FACE**

Pellevé Wrinkle Reduction System
is one of Rozina's favourite treatments
because she considers it safe, but highly
effective, with minimal side effects and
no recovery time.

It uses radiofrequency to heat up the
skin and tighten wrinkles on the jawline,
neck, cheeks and around the mouth and
eyes. Virtually painless, there is no need
for anaesthetic or skin cooling, meaning
the patient can describe the depth of
feeling to the practitioner to achieve the
best possible result. Energy is precisely
delivered to the skin's dermal layer
stimulating collagen production without
damage to the epidermis.

Occasionally patients will experience
mild redness or swelling but this usually
goes within hours and no recovery time
is necessary. And there are instant
results. There is an immediate
improvement in skin quality and
appearance, with a noticeable lift and
smoother tone. Two to three sessions
are recommended for the best results
after which patients look fresher and
younger. The effects are long lasting
if not permanent.

COST: £600+ PER FACE PER SESSION
(THREE RECOMMENDED).

Transderm Mesotherapy is a feel-
good treatment with instant results.
'This is the sort of pampering treatment
the stars indulge in pre-Oscars',
Rozina explained.

The Dermoelectroporation technology
uses low-energy electrical pulses to
allow large molecules (vitamins,
minerals, peptides, growth factors,
hyaluronic acid) to penetrate the skin
and rapidly enter the cells of the dermis
without the use of multiple injections.
This painless and pleasant treatment
nourishes and rejuvenates the
appearance of the skiin and promotes
improvement in quality and texture.

As well as face and neck treatment,
mesotherapy can also be used on the
backs of hands, buttocks and thighs,
reducing cellulite and stretch marks.
For optimum results, a course of
sessions is recommended.

COST: £200+ PER SESSION.

HOW
NOT
TO
GET
OLD
59
**TREATMENTS
FOR THE
FACE**

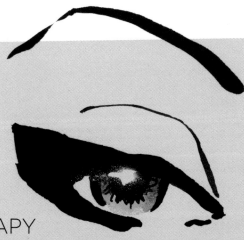

DRACULA THERAPY

S3 or Stimulated Self Serum Skin Therapy – more commonly known as Dracula or Vampire Therapy – was introduced to the UK by the London-based French doctor Daniel Sister.

In the treatment, blood is taken from the patient's arm and immediately centrifuged for five minutes to separate it into red blood cells, clear serum or plasma and platelets. Vitamins and amino acids are added to enrich the serum, which is then injected back into the forehead, cheeks, neck or back of the hand. It can also be used to treat dark under-eye circles. The serum is rich in growth factors and natural proteins that can repair cell damage and promote healing and regrowth. This stimulates the production of fibroblasts and collagen, resulting in greater skin elasticity and plumper, more youthful-looking skin. There should be a reduction in redness and the appearance of wrinkles and scarring.

After treatment the face will feel tender and there may be minimal swelling or bruising but no recovery time is needed. There is usually some immediate improvement but real effects appear over three to four weeks. Retreatments are recommended after four to six months.

Although new for the skin, it has been used for the past two decades by dentists to treat receding gums and in the US plasma is injected to ease sports' injuries.

COST: £500 PER SESSION.

HOW
NOT
TO
GET
OLD
60
**TREATMENTS
FOR THE
FACE**

EXPERT PROFILE
DR MAURICE DRAY

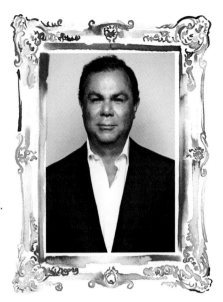

Dr Maurice Dray is a French dermatologist and gerontologist with over twenty-five years experience. He is a pioneer of cosmetic medicine with clinics in Paris and London.

In Dr Dray's lip treatment soft, natural hyaluronic gel is injected into the lips using an electronic syringe to give deep hydration, resulting in fuller, natural-looking lips.

The Ten-Minute Facelift is one of his most popular treatments. This is a non-invasive alternative to surgery, in particular firming the jawline and guarding against the development of jowls. The emphasis is on creating a subtle, fresh look and its many fans claim it keeps them looking younger longer. It is recommended from the age of thirty onwards.

The treatment begins with a fruit scrub and peel to remove any dead skin cells, followed by mesotherapy to hydrate skin and give it a vitamin boost, stimulating fibroblasts. Elastin, minerals, multivitamins and hyaluronic acid are injected in tiny pinpricks all over the face. Then the facelift proper begins.

Micro-particles of man-made chemicals called biphasic tricalcium phosphates (BTCPs) which are commonly used in dental powders, antacids and calcium supplements, are combined with hyaluronic acid gel and vitamins and injected under the chin, along the jawline and into the nasolabial, or marionette, lines. A syringe is used for the injections which take around ten minutes. Despite the use of anaesthetic cream, it has to be said they are painful. A deep, intense massage follows to make sure the fillers are evenly absorbed.

Using icepacks afterwards can help with any bruises, which should disappear completely in about a week, although they are easy to camouflage. There will be some immediate improvement to the skin as the hyaluronic acid takes effect, hydrating and plumping it.

The real results take up to eight weeks to show and last between ten and fifteen months. The BTCPs and hyaluronic acid biodegrade over time and collagen fibres develop, restoring volume and elasticity. Dr Dray recommends a course of three treatments six to eight months apart for maximum effect.

COST: £300 FOR LIP TREATMENT; £400 FOR 10-MINUTE FACELIFT.

HOW
NOT
TO
GET
OLD
61
**TREATMENTS
FOR THE
FACE**

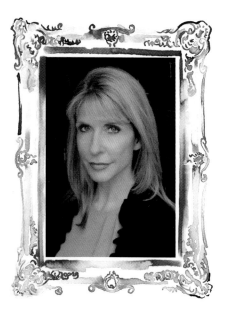

EXPERT PROFILE
DR TRACY MOUNTFORD

Dr Mountford MBBS, MBCAM was one of the first fully trained advanced cosmetic practitioners in the UK and is now one of the most respected doctors in the aesthetics industry. She has over twenty-three years experience in advanced non-surgical facial rejuvenation techniques, with a vast amount of expertise.

After qualifying as a doctor in 1985, Tracy initially worked as an anaesthetist. Always good with her hands, she is noted for her light touch, and after a stint working in the US she was inspired by the achievements she saw in non-surgical cosmetic medicine and changed career direction. She learned her craft and set up her own clinic, The Cosmetic Skin Clinic, with practices in Harley Street, London, and Buckinghamshire. She is one of the few doctors profiled in *Tatler's Beauty and Cosmetic Surgery Guide*, where she is described as a 'technical ace' and her clinic named 'Best for Fillers', so she has quite a reputation.

She prefers to think in terms of a 'make under'; the key is that it should not look like someone has had work done. 'I approach every patient as I would wish to be treated myself', Tracy explains.

Her treatments work to enhance natural beauty rather than changing a person's looks. Her trademark is a softening of lines and facial recontouring to enhance attractiveness and give a fresh airbrushed appearance, making everyone look as good as they can for their age.

HOW
NOT
TO
GET
OLD
62
TREATMENTS
FOR THE
FACE

SAHRAE'S STORY (PART ONE)

Now forty-four, Sahrae feels far older than her age. For all of her adult life she has no front teeth and is now having dental implants (see page 96). This has had a knock-on effect on her looks and so she has decided to address some of the other things that she feels are ageing, in particular her frown lines, hollow cheeks, the marionette lines between her mouth and chin and wrinkles around her mouth.

'All women have a natural beauty about them – my job is to bring that out', Tracy has said, and she immediately made Sahrae feel at ease.

For the first time, Sahrae felt that someone understood both what she wanted and actually made her feel that less was needed than she had thought. Dr Mountford was the first practitioner to make her feel attractive and to point out all her good features. It's not surprising that Sahrae opted to have her cosmetic treatments with Tracy.

THE TREATMENT

When Tracy first saw Sahrae, her immediate recommendation was that she stop using henna on her eyebrows, which were too dark and overly arched. 'Over elevated eyebrows are very ageing – you just need to look at your daughter to see what natural brows are like.' Tracy is very aware of keeping treatments appropriate to age. Very plump lips, for instance, can look wrong and artificial on older women.

Tracy suggested a combination of small amounts of Botox® and fillers to enhance Sahrae's looks and to soften the frown lines, nose-to-mouth, marionette and lip lines. Fillers will be used at the tops of the cheeks to give a little extra support and a lifting effect. Botox will be used to treat the brow lines, to lift the wrinkles around the eyes and to tighten the jawline and neck. Finally, radiofrequency skin tightening will provide extra lift to her jawline.

As the fillers are naturally biodegradable and Botox is not permanent, Sahrae will need maintenance. Normally Botox needs topping up two to three times a year and fillers every six to twelve months, depending on the patient.

No recovery time is needed after treatment, although care should be taken to remain upright for a few hours and there could be some bruising and slight swelling afterwards, depending on skin type.

GENERAL ADVICE

Tracy would always assess everyone's needs and preferences individually, but considers Botox and fillers to be the basic 'bread and butter' of anti-ageing treatments. In the hands of a skilled practitioner, she believes the incidence of side effects is rare; what marks out an expert is the knowledge and ability to rectify any reactions to a procedure. Her clinic sees around seventy patients a day and Tracy herself has worked with Botox for seventeen years. She stresses the need to avoid overuse,

'Faces are meant to move', and uses small amounts to achieve a natural youthful lift.

She suggests that as we age, skin benefits from hydrating, revitalizing treatments to attract water to the lower layers of the dermis and improve structure, firmness and elasticity. Fillers such as Juvederm Hydrate or Restylane Vital also help to stimulate the body's own ability to produce collagen, avoiding the development of further wrinkles.

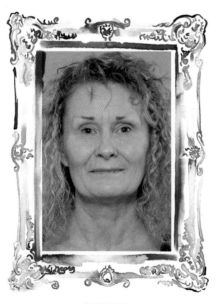

BEFORE

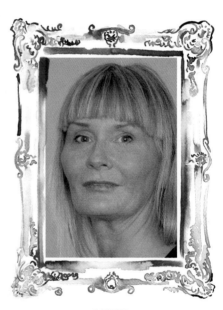

AFTER

HOW
NOT
TO
GET
OLD
64
**TREATMENTS
FOR THE
FACE**

BOTOX

Botulinum toxin is commercially available as Botox®, Dysport®, Azzalure® or Myobloc®. Botulinum toxin is a naturally occurring protein derived from the bacteria *clostridium botulinum*. It works by blocking a chemical responsible for muscle contraction, thereby temporarily paralysing muscles. As new nerves grow muscles are reactivated. Botox was first used in 1978 to treat eye spasms but it was not used cosmetically to smooth wrinkles until 1990.

It is used to lessen the appearance of wrinkles caused by muscle contractions such as forehead lines, frown lines and crows' feet, rather than those caused by sun damage or tissue sagging. Injections take just a few minutes and begin to take effect two to three days later, with full effects noticeable after one to two weeks, lasting between three and six months. Several injections are usually needed to treat an area and there can be localized bruising or discomfort, but no recovery period is needed.

Botox is still the most popular anti-ageing treatment with 2.5 million men and women using it in the UK, France, Italy, Germany and Spain. The trend is for little and often to create a more subtle natural look. When used well by qualified and experienced practitioners who really know what they're doing, there's no doubt it can delay the signs of ageing. But overuse may lead to resistance to treatment, muscle weakness or an exaggeration of facial asymmetry. A slight drooping of the eyelid can sometimes occur after injections above the eyebrows which usually wears off and can be helped by eye drops.

COST: £200–£300 PER AREA TREATED.

EXPERT ADVICE

Avoid bending or lying down for 3–4 hours after Botox injections and avoid rubbing the area for 12–24 hours.

HOW
NOT
TO
GET
OLD
65
**TREATMENTS
FOR THE
FACE**

THE LONG-TERM EFFECTS OF BOTOX

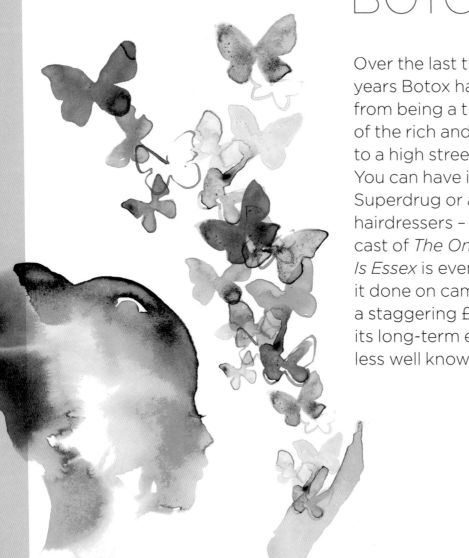

Over the last twenty years Botox has gone from being a treatment of the rich and famous, to a high street commodity. You can have it done in Superdrug or at your local hairdressers – and the cast of *The Only Way Is Essex* is even having it done on camera. Worth a staggering £18 million, its long-term effects are less well known.

But did you know that Botox originally came from a sausage? It was first discovered in 1820 by Justinus Kerner, a German doctor. He named it botulinum toxin, from the Latin meaning 'sausage poison', shortened to 'Botox'. In the 1940s it was discovered that Botox could stop communication between nerves and muscles and its first medical use was in the 1970s to stop facial spasms. In 1987 a Canadian ophthalmologist noticed that Botox could also smooth out the glabellar frown lines on the face, and Botox for cosmetic purposes was born.

Botox is a controversial treatment, and many have questioned the long term effects of its use. One issue is that some practitioners are suggesting that young people, without any obvious wrinkles, should have Botox to prevent future signs of ageing. Doctor Darren McKowen, a plastic surgeon, has refused to inject patients as young as nineteen, arguing that young people should not have Botox because of the atrophying or wasting effect it has on muscles, and that in the long run it can make users look much older. Shockingly, the youngest ever user is just eight years old, with injections given to her by her beautician mother!

A preliminary study carried out by scientists at the University of Munich, and published in the Journal for Dermatologic Surgery, found that muscle atrophy of the face caused by Botox lasted for up to twelve months, a considerable length of time after the wrinkles it was used to treat had returned. The researchers injected two men who had never had Botox before, once in the muscle of their foreheads. The men had MRI scans at various intervals for the next twelve months. They found there was a 46–48 per cent reduction in the muscle volume up to twelve months after the injection. The scientists' conclusion was that further research should be conducted into the effects of Botox on muscle atrophy, as it seems that even after it has been reabsorbed by the body, muscles continue to atrophy.

Doctor Nicholas Lowe, who carried out one of the earliest clinical studies of Botox for cosmetic purposes, and was the first to inject it in the UK, believes a little muscle atrophy can be a desirable thing, but he too is shocked by the number of young people being treated. He is also shocked by the frequency with which people have Botox injections – he has used it for the last twenty-two years but only has a treatment once a year. He cites instances of clinics that send out reminder text messages to their clients after just three months.

Botox has many medical uses, and its cosmetic effects cannot be denied. However, it is recommended you should not have Botox until you are at least thirty, or after wrinkles have begun to appear, and then it should not be used too often. It is worth being aware that, despite the fact that there have been a number of clinical studies, it is still a comparatively new medicine for which the long-term effects remain relatively unknown.

HOW
NOT
TO
GET
OLD
67
**TREATMENTS
FOR THE
FACE**

INTENSE PULSED LIGHT

Commonly abbreviated to IPL, this is used for skin rejuvenation and healing. Different from a laser, light therapy penetrates deep into the skin to boost cell energy, stimulating fibroblast activity and collagen production. It helps to correct skin blemishes, acne scars and rosacea, and reduces the appearance of wrinkles, red spider veins and uneven pigmentation. It smoothes skin tone and leaves the skin firmer and more radiant. It can also be used to treat facial (and body) hair.

Up to eight treatments may be needed for hair removal, usually a month to six weeks apart. For age spots and red veins typically three to five sessions are necessary, carried out a month to six weeks apart.

COST: ABOUT £100 PER SESSION.

MICRODERMABRASION

A hand-held device targets a jet of micro crystals at the face and neck which are then vacuumed away, taking the top layer of dead skin cells with them. The crystals effectively exfoliate, improving tone and texture and revealing newer, softer skin. At the same time, collagen production is stimulated. This relatively painless treatment reduces the appearance of fine lines and scars, sun damage, age spots and large pores. Following microdermabrasion, skin will respond better to anti-ageing creams.

There's a very low risk of scarring or uneven pigmentation in comparison with other resurfacing treatments and no recovery time is needed, although skin may be red for a few hours afterwards. A course of five to ten treatments is usually recommended depending on skin damage and the results you want to achieve.

COST: FROM £65 PER SESSION.

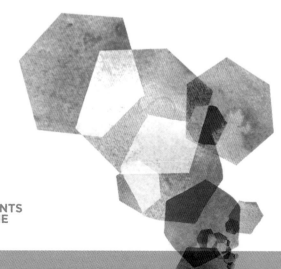

HOW
NOT
TO
GET
OLD
68
**TREATMENTS
FOR THE
FACE**

CHEMICAL PEELS

These are among the most popular non-invasive treatments for rejuvenating the skin. They are used to improve texture and reduce the appearance of fine lines and wrinkles, uneven pigmentation and sun damage, and to treat acne, acne scars and rosacea.

AHA PEELS Alpha hydroxy acids such as glycolic, lactic or fruit acids are natural substances that have been used for centuries to boost the complexion. They vary in strength from 5 per cent concentrations which can be used at home, salon strength which are 20–40 per cent, to intense, medical-strength 70–90 per cent peels which should only ever be used by fully trained doctors or nurses. Initially skin looks as if it is severely sunburned, then after two to three days it begins to peel. The length of time taken to peel completely and recover depends on the depth of the peel but the effects should last for about a year. Stronger peels should not be performed more than once a year. After treatment it's important to take extra care in the sun, wearing a sunblock with an SPF 30.

COST: FROM £100.

TCA PEELS Trichloroacetic acid is a medium- to deep-peeling agent usually used in a 10–35 per cent concentration. It can be painful as the top layer of the skin is removed and stronger solutions may penetrate deeper into the dermis. As the damaged skin layers peel away, the healing process stimulates cell growth and collagen production, resulting in new, healthier, younger-looking skin.

A course of one to three treatments carried out a month apart is usually recommended and recovery from each treatment can take up to a week. Skin should be protected and moisturized with a thin layer of Vaseline. As with AHA peels, it's vital to be extra vigilant in the sun, protecting with an SPF 30.

COST: MILDER PEELS FROM £100;
FULL TCA PEELS UP TO £700.

HOW
NOT
TO
GET
OLD
69
**TREATMENTS
FOR THE
FACE**

LASER SKIN RESURFACING

A variety of laser systems are now available including carbon dioxide and fractional lasers. In particular they are used to treat the effects of sun damage, uneven pigmentation, fine lines around the mouth, eyes and on the cheeks, rough skin and acne scars.

Results can be long-lasting but this is a serious procedure and patients need a local anaesthetic for small areas or a general anaesthetic if the whole face is treated. Skin is very red and raw after treatment. Initial healing usually takes between seven and ten days but the newly exposed skin is red for two to six months. Sun exposure during this time should be avoided as it increases the risk of pigmentation changes – either darkening or lightening of skin. If a patient has previously suffered from cold sores they can recur, so preventative treatment will be needed.

COST: FROM £2,500.

NON-SURGICAL FACELIFT

Lasers can also be used for non-surgical facelifts. The procedure takes about one and a half hours and the face is anaesthetized first. Microlaser resurfacing and fractional lasers are used to effectively burn the surface layer of skin – anyone considering this procedure should be aware there is a distinct smell of burning during treatment.

Afterwards, skin will be bright red, while the eye area, which has been protected, will look white and puffy. Skin must be treated as if burned and constantly covered with moisturizer. The surface layers will peel away to expose new skin, removing fine lines and the effects of sun damage. As with all laser treatments there is a risk of infection as there will be open wounds, and a danger of scarring and pigmentation. There will also be a certain amount of pain and discomfort. But with an expert practitioner, the right aftercare and good healing, the newly exposed skin looks fresher and younger.

COST: ABOUT £4,000.

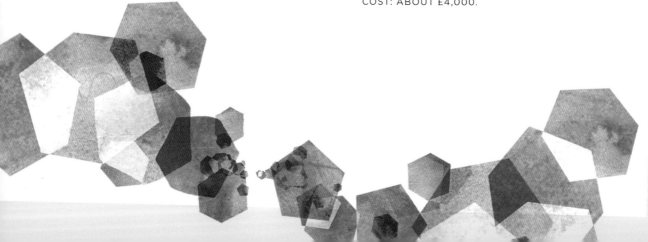

EXPERT PROFILE
DR RITA RAKUS

Dubbed 'The London Lip Queen', Dr Rita Rakus has been in the cosmetic industry for over twenty years, specializing in non-invasive cosmetic procedures to treat the signs of facial and body ageing. She qualified as a medical practitioner at Sydney University in Australia and now runs the largest solo non-surgical practice in the UK.

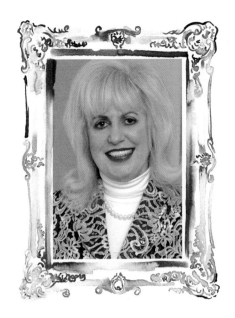

Ultherapy uses ultrasound to stimulate the deep structural support layers of the skin, encouraging the production of new collagen to strengthen and tone the skin over time from within. It gives a short-term boost but the real results develop over the next two to three months. Ultrasound imaging allows Rita to see where energy is being delivered to make sure it will have the most effect.

It is typically used on the brow line, for sagging skin on eyelids, neck and the jaw and is most effective for those with 'mild to moderate skin laxity'. Most people need only one treatment and results last up to a year or longer, depending on a patient's natural ageing, after which touch-up treatments can maintain improvements.

Ultherapy to tighten the jawline typically takes 30–45 minutes. There can be some discomfort during the procedure and afterwards some redness and slight swelling. Bruising can also develop but is unusual. After the treatment it is important to avoid extremes of heat and cold and to use sunblock, as well as non-irritating products for 24 hours.

Immediately after the Ulthera procedure, skin will feel smoother and younger. Over the next weeks the jawline will look tighter and more defined.

COST: FROM £1,200 FOR PARTIAL FACE, INCLUDING JAWLINE; £4,000 FOR FULL FACE AND NECK.

HOW
NOT
TO
GET
OLD
71
**TREATMENTS
FOR THE
FACE**

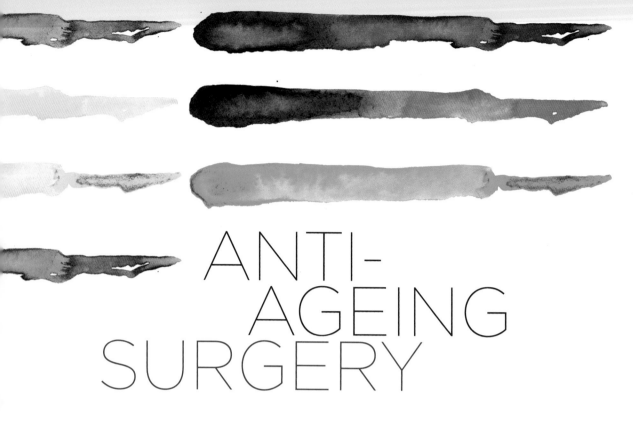

ANTI-AGEING SURGERY

Rajiv Grover, president of the BAAPS said, 'Whilst there is an undeniable rise in demand for non-surgical treatments of the face, for example Botox and fillers, once there is actual loose skin in the neck or jowling, only surgery is likely to make a significant improvement and the public seem to be increasingly aware of this.'

EXPERT PROFILE
BARRY JONES
CONSULTANT PLASTIC AND CRANIOFACIAL SURGEON

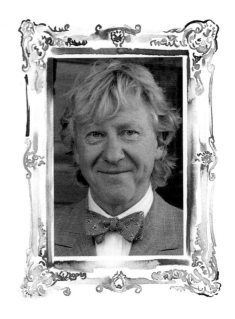

Barry Jones began his medical training at the University of London and then in craniofacial, reconstructive, plastic and aesthetic surgery in London, Paris and the US. His interest in plastic surgery developed from his craniofacial experience and from working at Mount Vernon Hospital in London in the plastic surgery unit, at a time when microsurgery was very new. He now works at King Edward VII Hospital and Great Ormond Street Hospital and has a private clinic on Upper Wimpole Street, London.

Mr Jones' advice to anyone considering plastic surgery is to choose your surgeon very carefully and look at their body of work to see what their specific interests are. He will always listen carefully to what the patient wants but feels it is important to make sure patients are realistic about what can be achieved. He tries to adapt his facelifts to the individual and takes pride in his natural results.

Around the age of fifty is the most common time for facelifts to be carried out but the range is anything from forty to ninety. 'The right time is when it's right for the individual', Barry stresses.

Normal ageing obviously continues after surgery and he has recently published a paper called *How Long Does a Facelift Last*. He collected data from a large group of his patients over a ten-year period, comparing photographs taken in the same studio, with the same lights and camera, using both subjective analysis and a computer programme which enabled the changes that occurred in fixed points on the face to be measured over time.

A short summary of the detailed findings were that after five and a half years, 78 per cent of patients still looked better than they had done before their facelifts. The study continues and it appears that many of these improvements will last for much longer periods.

HOW
NOT
TO
GET
OLD
73
**TREATMENTS
FOR THE
FACE**

FACELIFTS

FACELIFTS are most effective when the skin and muscles of the face and neck have begun to sag but skin still retains some elasticity and the underlying bone structure is well defined. For this reason most are carried out on patients aged forty to sixty, although they can be successful on people in their eighties.

A GOOD FACELIFT should take years off your age without it being obvious that you've had any work done. But this is a very complicated operation with side effects including damage to facial nerves, loss of feeling and blood clots. As with any surgery, it's vital to do your research and choose a fully qualified surgeon with lots of experience in the procedure. This will reduce the risks and should ensure a good, natural-looking result.

THE PROCEDURE is carried out in hospital, usually under general anaesthetic – it's a long operation but it is possible to opt for local anaesthetic and sedation. Incisions follow the natural creases in front of the ears and extend into the hairline above and behind the ears. It is sometimes necessary to make an incision under the chin to remove fat from the jawline and chin by liposuction.

FACELIFTS WORK BEST for the lower half of the face, particularly the jawline and neck. To lift a wrinkled forehead, sagging eyebrows or loose skin around the eyes, you would need to consider an endoscopic brow lift or eyelid reduction. It is possible to combine all three. Other extras that could be done at the same time are cheek, chin and lip enhancements.

SOMETIMES ONLY THE SKIN IS LIFTED, but more often the underlying muscle is also lifted, although sutured separately. Drains may be inserted and the face is usually bandaged to minimize swelling and bruising. These remain for one or two days and sutures are removed after seven to eight days.

YOU SHOULD EXPECT BRUISING and puffiness. Your face may also feel rather stiff. A degree of numbness is also not unusual and should disappear within a few weeks or months.

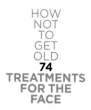

These are some of the different types of facelift procedures most commonly carried out:

MINI-FACELIFT This uses shorter incisions, thereby minimizing scars and generally reducing recovery times. There are various techniques including MACS (minimal access cranial suspension), S-lift and Thread lift. S-shaped incisions are made around the ear, halving the length of the scars. They don't have such dramatic results but the effects last as long as classic facelifts.

ONE-STITCH OR SILHOUETTE FACELIFT This uses innovative Silhouette Sutures®, which are not barbed and so prevent damage to the surrounding tissue. Small incisions are hidden in the hairline at the side of the forehead through which threads are gently passed. The Silhouette Sutures are made from polypropylene, a biocompatible material which has been used for many years in cardiovascular and ophthalmic surgery. These work using small, resorbable cones which anchor themselves in deep tissue, resulting in tension which lifts sagging tissue. Over time, new tissue forms around these cones which dissolve, leaving the skin and new tissue anchored in place.

DEEP FACELIFT This is carried out endoscopically and usually at an earlier age than a standard facelift. It tightens the middle part of the face and lifts the outer angle of the eyes, reducing crows' feet. Incisions are made beneath the eyelashes of the lower eyelids and sometimes in the upper gum line.

COST: £1500–£2,500 FOR A ONE-STITCH FACELIFT; FROM £2000–£10,000 FOR A MINI-LIFT; FROM £6000 FOR A FULL FACELIFT.

BROW LIFT

A brow lift literally lifts the skin on the forehead and sometimes the muscles below, tightening everything to remove wrinkles and sagging, leaving the face looking younger, softer and less fraught. If overdone, it can result in that odd, startled expression where eyebrows look too high. Usually performed endoscopically through keyhole surgery, a few small staples or studs are left in the hairline. These are either removed or dissolve over time. Bruising around the eyes spreads down into the face but should fade after a week to ten days.

COST: FROM £1,500.

EYELID SURGERY

Eyelid surgery, or blepharoplasty, is a procedure to remove fat, usually along with excess skin and muscle, from the upper and lower eyelids. In a typical procedure, the surgeon makes incisions following the natural lines of the eyelids – in the creases of upper lids and just below the lashes in the lower lids. These incisions are extended a little way into the crow's feet at the corners of the eyes. Surplus fat, excess skin and sagging muscle are then removed.

The surgery will not remove or tighten wrinkles around the eyes unless they are part of the skin which is removed. Any scarring is usually well hidden but post-operative complications can include dry eyes caused by tear duct damage, and if too much skin is removed it can be difficult to shut the eyes properly. Recovery time is usually a week to ten days.

COST: ABOUT £3,000 FOR UPPER OR LOWER EYELID SURGERY; £4,400 FOR BOTH.

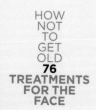
HOW
NOT
TO
GET
OLD
76
**TREATMENTS
FOR THE
FACE**

EXPERT
ADVICE BEFORE AND AFTER SURGERY

BEFORE…

◎ If you're planning to lose weight it's best to do so before the surgery.

◎ Avoid any medication containing aspirin or anti-inflammatories for at least two weeks before the procedure.

◎ You should also stop smoking at least two weeks beforehand to avoid complications and delayed recovery.

◎ Plan for hair treatments including colouring before your operation, as scars will be sensitive to chemicals for some weeks.

AFTER…

◎ You should expect to take two weeks off work, with complete rest for a week.

◎ It's vital to keep blood pressure down. The easy rule to remember is to keep head above heart at all times, which includes sleeping propped up for at least ten days and two weeks if possible.

◎ Both smoking and alcohol are a very bad idea and should be avoided during recovery.

◎ Don't take ibuprofen, aspirin or any anti-inflammatories including fish oils and vitamin E.

◎ Paracetamol can help ease discomfort.

◎ Avoid strenuous sport, saunas and massage for at least six weeks but always check with your surgeon.

◎ Most people return to work and normal social activities after two weeks.

◎ Make-up can help cover bruising.

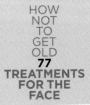

HOW
NOT
TO
GET
OLD
77
**TREATMENTS
FOR THE
FACE**

MARION'S STORY

Marion lost her sense of taste three years ago after brain surgery and as a result lost over 30 kilos in weight, dropping from a size 18 to a size 8. The extreme weight loss has left her with excess skin and deep-set wrinkles. 'I've got the figure of a twenty-year-old and the face of a sixty-year-old', and when Marion tells people her real age she knows they usually don't believe her. She has been mistaken for a sixty-seven-year old and just wants to look her real age of forty-seven.

'I feel as though I lost "me" and all my confidence along with the weight', Marion explained. Friends who haven't seen her since before the weight loss think she looks exhausted.

Exercise has helped tone her legs and body but has made no difference to her bingo wings and boobs. Eventually she would like to treat them, too, but feels that her face is her priority as she can't hide it behind clothes.

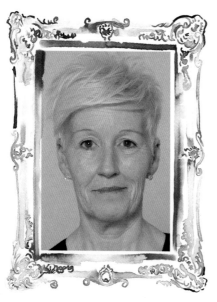

BEFORE

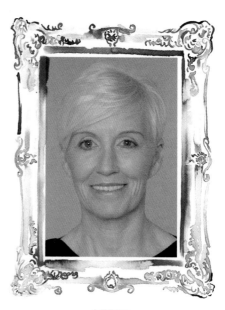

AFTER

HOW
NOT
TO
GET
OLD
78
TREATMENTS
FOR THE
FACE

EXPERT PROFILE
TAIMUR SHOAIB

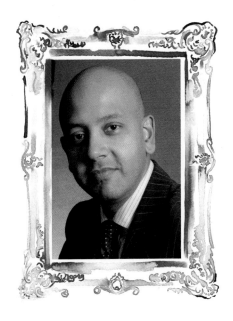

Practising at the Nuffield Hospital and Glasgow Royal Infirmary, Taimur Shoaib has seven years' experience as a consultant plastic surgeon. He enjoys the challenge that the precision and expertise of plastic surgery demands and likes making a difference to people's lives. His approach really appealed to Marion when she was considering surgery.

Mr Shoaib always tries to be realistic and guide patients on the best procedures to help them achieve what they want.

THE TREATMENT

It was decided that the most effective course was a full facelift with lipofilling to Marion's cheeks (taking fat from her stomach), an upper and lower eyelid blepharoplasty and laser treatments to improve the texture and tone of her skin. All the procedures would be done at the same time under local anaesthetic and sedation.

Immediately afterwards Marion's eyes will be swollen which could make it quite hard to see. The stitches for her facelift and her upper and lower eyelids will be taken out after five days.

She will stay in a hotel in Glasgow for a week's recuperation afterwards. As she lives in Birmingham she will not be able to fly for at least two weeks or travel at all immediately. This was a consideration but Marion was certain that Mr Shoaib was the best surgeon for her even though it meant travelling and staying away from home.

Because of the laser treatment, the skin must be kept moist at all times with Vaseline or similar.

HOW
NOT
TO
GET
OLD
79
TREATMENTS
FOR THE
FACE

CHINS AND CHEEKS

COSMETIC SURGERY can reshape chins which either jut out too much or are too recessive. Surgery can also add extra definition to cheekbones. Problems with jaw size as a whole or misalignment of teeth would be referred to a maxillo-facial surgeon.

CHIN BONE can be shaved down to correct a jutting chin while implants would be inserted to plump out flat cheekbones or recessive chins. Implants are usually made from silicone or another non-biological material. Occasionally the bone can be advanced or moved forward to give the chin more projection. For chins, incisions are made in the groove between the lower lip and gum, while for cheeks cuts are usually made inside the mouth where the cheek meets the upper gum.

SCARRING should be minimal but you should expect bruising and some swelling for up to three weeks. Numbness of the upper lip and side of the nose is not unusual, sometimes followed by pins and needles.

IMPLANTS IN THE CHIN can occasionally slip, requiring a further operation. They can also weaken teeth if roots are nearby. It is a good idea to have a thorough dental check-up before chin or cheek surgery.

COST: FROM £4,000.

EXPERT ADVICE
AFTERCARE

◎ Be very gentle with your face.

◎ Take at least a week off work.

◎ Avoid the temptation to feel or move an implant and don't rest your chin on your hands.

◎ Be scrupulous about oral hygiene but go easy with the toothbrush. Use a mouthwash after meals, especially while stitches are dissolving.

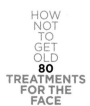

ANN'S STORY

Ann, 49, is from Lancashire. She lost a staggering 18 stone in weight after having a gastrectomy in 2010 and is now a healthy size 14. She had expected excess skin on her body and arms but an unwelcome side effect of the weight loss was loose, sagging skin on her face and neck leaving her looking a lot older.

She has tried Botox® and in fact confesses to having probably too much, topping up every ten weeks; she has also had fillers in her chin. But now her weight is stable, she is looking for a permanent solution. With a slim silhouette, Ann feels younger overall but thinks her face aged twenty years as the weight fell away. 'I now want to look as glam as I feel.'

Ann had already heard of her surgeon, Alex Karidis, before deciding she needed a facelift. She had seen him featured in various magazines and on television, and been impressed with his work.

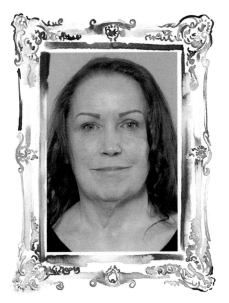

BEFORE

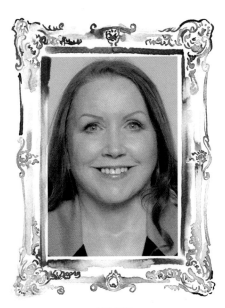

AFTER

HOW
NOT
TO
GET
OLD
81
TREATMENTS
FOR THE
FACE

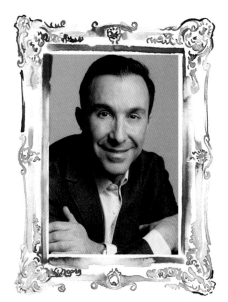

EXPERT PROFILE
ALEX KARIDIS

One of the UK's most well-known and respected cosmetic surgeons, Alex Karidis has over twenty-five years' experience in plastic surgery and has run his own practice in St John's Wood, London for sixteen years. He performs an average of 150 facial lifts a year, including brown and mid-face lifts.

He has always been interested in the idea of correcting people's external issues. Experienced in a wide range of surgeries, he believes the challenge with faces is to identify exactly what it is that a patient does not like about their appearance or wants to change. He will offer an opinion but for him the key is to know what a patient wants, so that he can then guide them towards the right treatment.

Mr Karidis always encourages potential patients to read widely, so they can be as clear and informed as possible about their options. He shows patients lots of photos of his work, 'I like to make sure they have a flavour of what I can do and a clear notion of my aesthetic sense. It is important their ideas are in tune with mine.'

Alex Karidis feels there are more options now than ever before when it comes to anti-ageing treatments. When asked what you can do to avoid surgery it is no surprise that he cites the obvious culprits: smoking and the sun. However, he suggests that access to many non-surgical procedures including Botox, dermal fillers, lasers and mechanical devices to deliver effective treatments deep into the dermis can all work to hold back the most obvious signs of ageing when applied correctly. And he firmly believes there's no point advocating something you would not do yourself – he has had Botox and dermal fillers from time to time and has done over his career in the industry. He is also a strong advocate of good basic skincare, most importantly moisturizing.

For those to whom something drastic has happened, or for whom ageing is accelerating, or where non-surgical procedures are no longer enough, a facelift, although invasive, can offer dramatic results.

HOW
NOT
TO
GET
OLD
82
TREATMENTS
FOR THE
FACE

THE TREATMENT

Ann has opted for a lower facelift, with microliposuction to her chin and neck to remove fat and a light endowbrow lift. She is not having any work to her lower eyelids as there is insufficient loose skin and the end result would be too tight.

The whole operation will take about three hours and Ann will spend two nights in hospital. As there will be no stitches around her eyes all stitches will be dissolvable.

★ As well as the usual recommendations for post-facelift surgery, including keeping her head elevated and sleeping well propped up, Ann has been given arnica to aid healing.

★ She also has cold compress ice packs to apply for 15 minutes every hour after the surgery.

★ She has been advised to wash her hair very carefully with baby shampoo every day to guard against infection, afterwards drying with a low-heat hair dryer to keep scars dry.

★ Bath water must be no more than tepid.

★ She must use factor 50 suncream in the sun – forever.

★ Everyone heals at a different rate but swelling usually takes two to three weeks to go down.

★ She should be 'restaurant-ready' with make-up to camouflage after four weeks.

★ It can take six months for the full effects and the 'new' face to be fully apparent.

COST: £14,900, INCLUDING HOSPITAL FEES AND ALL TESTS.

HOW
NOT
TO
GET
OLD
83
**TREATMENTS
FOR THE
FACE**

NOSES

It's a myth that noses grow as we age but as your face thins and skin sags your nose can appear bigger. Surgery to reshape, increase or decrease the size is very common. A reduction rhinoplasty reduces the size and an augmentation rhinoplasty increases it.

REDUCTION RHINOPLASTY In a reduction rhinoplasty the bridge of the nose is usually broken and cartilage and bone are filed to reshape it. Cartilage around the nostrils can be moved to reshape the tip. The level of scarring varies and if it's possible to carry out the surgery internally there may be no visible scars. There is always some swelling and bruising especially around the eyes, which can take up to three months to go down completely. Initially you would also need to wear a splint but usually after three weeks you should stop looking as though you have just had surgery.

There are limits to what can be done in terms of age, elasticity of skin, any previous injury and the proportions of other features. You should be very clear about what you hope to achieve and discuss the procedure in detail with your surgeon. Patients can have difficulty breathing through the nose for the first week, and occasionally this is permanent.

AUGMENTATION RHINOPLASTY In an augmentation rhinoplasty an implant is used to rebuild the framework of the nose. This can be made from bone, cartilage or manufactured material. Bone is taken from the hip, rib or sometimes elbow, and cartilage from the ear or spare cartilage from inside the nose. Skin grafts can sometimes also be necessary.

Small implants can sometimes be inserted under local anaesthetic but larger operations using bone grafts would mean a longer stay in hospital. Further surgery can be necessary if there is infection or if an implant shifts, usually following an injury. Swelling and bruising should subside after a couple of weeks but it will be at least three months before the new shape properly matures.

COSTS: FROM £2,000, BUT PRICES VARY ACCORDING TO THE AMOUNT OF WORK DONE.

HOW
NOT
TO
GET
OLD
84
TREATMENTS
FOR THE
FACE

EXPERT
ADVICE
DR ROZINA ALI – EFFECTIVE ANTI-AGEING PROCEDURES

'I am a huge proponent of self-improvement. Sometimes well-thought-out surgery can redirect a whole life.' When asked for her advice on the most effective anti-ageing procedures for the face, Rozina concentrated on three main areas:

◎ TISSUES SAGE AS WE AGE Lipofilling – where your own fat is purified and then injected deep into cheeks and temples – can add volume and a youthful plumpness to the contours of your face.

◎ EYES CAN GET LOST and appear smaller as the delicate skin on eyelids crinkles and sags. Eyelid surgery, or blepharoplasty, is a relatively cost-effective surgery that really delivers results. Eyes appear open and younger, making you look more direct and powerful.

◎ IF WIDE EYES make you look warm and approachable, it's your mouth that suggests ageless sexiness. Lips thin and gums recede – sadly the expression 'long-in-the-tooth' has its origins in reality. However, kissable, full lips are possible at any age with the careful use of temporary hyaluronic acid (HA) fillers. Fat does not stay around the mouth and permanent collagen fillers should be avoided at all costs.

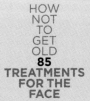

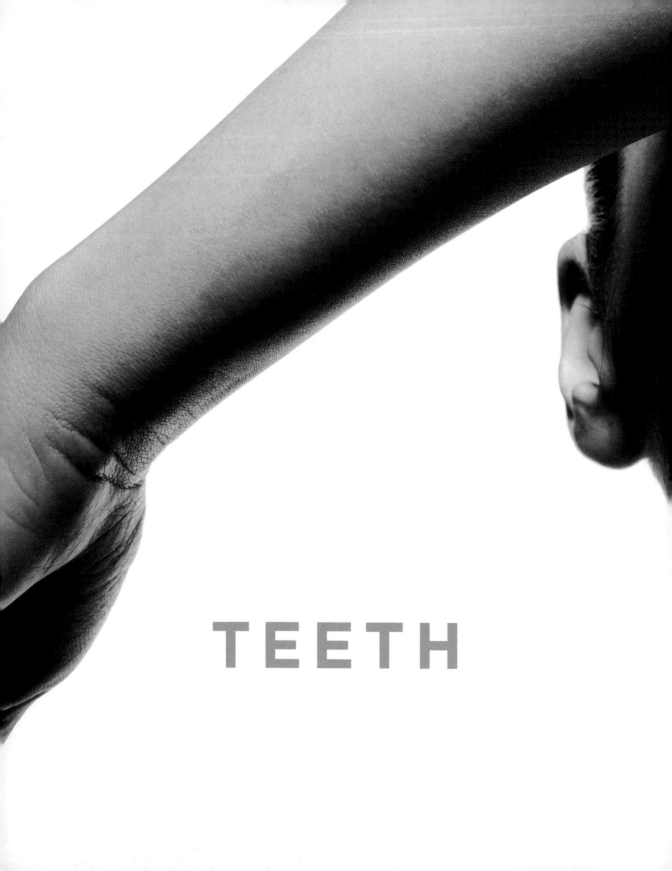

TEETH

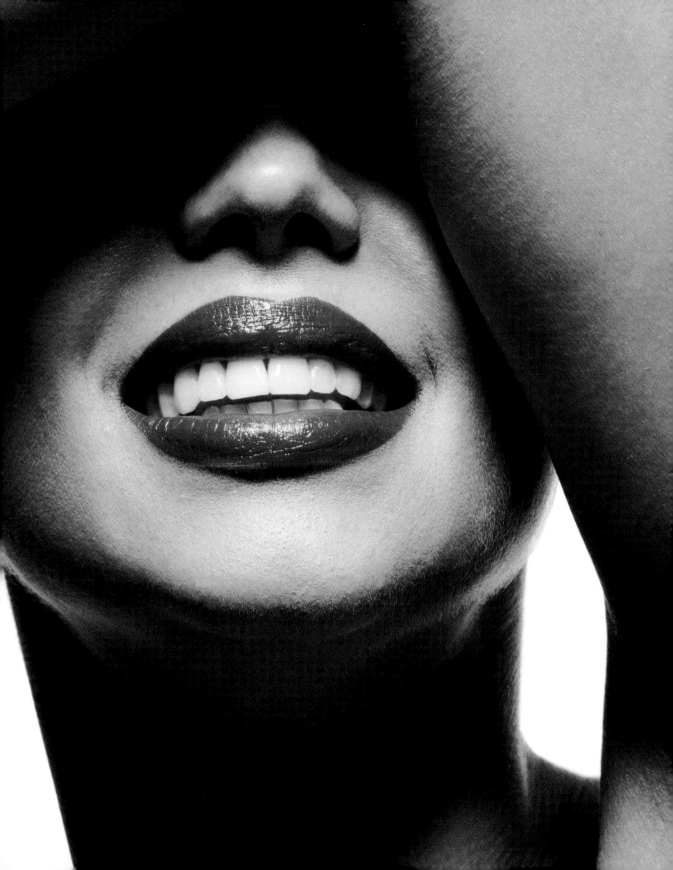

As you age teeth begin to dull and 'halo' shapes can develop at the edges of the tooth which can become very discoloured, making teeth look older. The shape of your face can also be affected as teeth wear down. Good oral hygiene and regular visits to the dentist are vital and it's important to maintain a healthy, balanced diet to ensure you receive all the nutrients you need, including calcium and vitamin D – both of which are essential for strong, healthy teeth.

Signs of ageing:
◎ Gums shrink and lose their shape.
◎ Receding gums add to the appearance of age, giving a 'long-in-the-tooth' effect.
◎ Bleeding, puffy gums and bad breath can all be symptoms of gum disease.
◎ Lips are also affected, especially if you're a smoker, with puckered lines, known as periodontal wrinkles, appearing around the contours of the mouth.

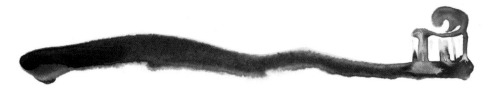

SIMPLE STEPS FOR A HEALTHY, YOUTHFUL SMILE

◎ BRUSH TEETH at least twice a day for two minutes. Whether you are using manual or electric, it's most important to choose a toothbrush that you'll use properly.

◎ CHOOSE SOFT-BRISTLED BRUSHES with a small head that fits inside your mouth so you can reach all areas.

◎ IT'S TIME TO BUY a new toothbrush when the bristles become splayed or start looking worn – usually every three months. However, if you have gum disease it's best to change after four to six weeks.

◎ ALWAYS CHANGE YOUR TOOTHBRUSH if you've been ill.

◎ USE TOOTHPASTE THAT CONTAINS FLOURIDE – a mineral that helps prevent tooth decay in people of all ages.

◎ WHITENING TOOTHPASTES contain carbamide peroxide like all toothpastes, but they may have additional polishing agents and chemicals that work more effectively against stains. They are ideal for smokers and tea, coffee and red wine drinkers.

◎ FLOSS at least once a day to remove food debris from the areas where your toothbrush can't reach and to prevent the build-up of plaque.

◎ WHEN USING A MOUTHWASH, look for one that's alcohol-free and contains fluoride.

◎ DENTAL HYGIENISTS can advise on oral hygiene as well as scaling teeth to remove tartar or calcium deposits.

◎ EVEN IF you have no obvious issues with your teeth you should visit your dentist for a check-up every six months to prevent any problems developing.

◎ BAD BREATH is most often caused by gum disease, cavities or poor oral hygiene. Prevent it by brushing twice a day (including the tongue), flossing, using a mouthwash, having regular dental check-ups and drinking plenty of water.

◎ A BALANCED DIET can really help you delay the signs of dental ageing. Vitamin D and calcium are essential for the development and maintenance of strong healthy teeth and Vitamin C helps fight infection.

THIS WORKS
It's not always practical to brush your teeth after eating something acidic or sweet but finishing with some hard cheese will reduce the damage and remove any harmful residue.

EXPERT ADVICE

It's not just your teeth and appearance that benefit from flossing – your heart will be healthier, too. A Swedish medical study found a link between gum disease, heart attacks and strokes. It seems the bacteria responsible for causing gum disease can trigger an immune response in the body leading to inflammation, including inflammation of the arteries.

THINGS TO AVOID...

◎ DON'T SMOKE In terms of appearance it stains teeth and causes periodontal lines around the mouth. It's also a disaster for oral health, depleting Vitamin C and other nutrients, and leaving you at greater risk of infection, gum disease and oral cancer.

◎ RESTRICT THE AMOUNT OF FIZZY DRINKS you have. The acid in carbon dioxide attacks tooth enamel, encouraging bacteria and decay.

◎ ALTHOUGH FRUIT JUICE may seem like a healthy option it's not great for teeth. The acid and fruit sugars in fruit juice can all cause damage.

◎ DARK-COLOURED FOODS and drinks uch as red wine, tea and coffee can all stain and discolour teeth making you look older. A whitening toothpaste can help keep staining at bay.

◎ CUT OUT SUGARY FOODS as well as drinks. They also attack enamel, promoting the growth of bacteria. Chewy or boiled sweets are particularly bad as they remain in your mouth for a long time, prolonging the attack on your teeth.

◎ YOU CAN HELP REDUCE DAMAGE by brushing your teeth twenty minutes after eating to allow your mouth's pH level to return to normal.

THIS WORKS
Regular flossing can knock six years off your apparent age according to US anti-ageing guru Dr Michael Roizen.

HOLDING BACK THE YEARS

Any procedure that improves the overall look of your teeth and smile is regarded as cosmetic dentistry. There is also an increasing trend for dental practices to offer facial rejuvenation treatments including Botox and fillers. As with any procedure, you should always check that your dentist is fully qualified and experienced. Personal recommendations are always reassuring but there are some questions you should ask as a safeguard.

Your checklist
◎ How many years have they been in practice?
◎ How many similar procedures have they carried out?
◎ Do they have a portfolio showing examples of their work?
◎ Do they offer any guarantees?
◎ Are follow-up checks and aftercare included?

TEETH WHITENING

The most popular of all cosmetic dental procedures, teeth whitening is not a new idea. The ancient Romans are known to have used a mixture of goat's milk and urea to bleach their teeth. Today, there are three main methods: the tray system which uses trays specially designed by your dentist to fit snugly over your teeth which you use at home; power whitening at the dentist's surgery using a light or laser; and DIY home bleaching kits which you buy over the counter from a chemist.

DIY HOME BLEACHING KITS

These work on the same principle as the dentist's tray method, but the tray is a standard size and not specifically moulded to fit your teeth. This means that the gel can leak and burn gums or cause mouth ulcers. The concentrations of bleach are also insufficient to achieve very satisfactory results.

COST: FROM £10.

THE TRAY AT-HOME WHITENING SYSTEM

This is the method the British Dental Health Federation recommends as the most effective and safest. Your dentist takes impressions of your teeth and customized trays are made up in a laboratory. At home you then apply hydrogen peroxide gel to the trays and wear them for an hour or two a day for ten to fourteen days, depending on how white you want your teeth to be. This is a gentle, easy system which is known to work and results can last up to three years. Legislation passed in November 2012 in the UK limited the concentration of carbamide peroxide used to 18 per cent, the equivalent of 6 per cent hydrogen peroxide.

COST: £300-£700.

VENEERS

LIGHT OR LASER POWER WHITENING

This can only be done in a dental surgery. Lips and gums are first coated with silicon for protection, then a concentrated bleaching gel is applied to the teeth, after which a high-intensity light is shone onto them. There are usually three concurrent twenty-minute applications. The heat activates the peroxide which penetrates the enamel and bleaches stains. The results are instant and last up to three years. However, many dentists will advise against this treatment as it does cause some damage to the enamel – roughly equivalent to drinking half a can of fizzy drink.

COST: £700–£1,300.

A thin layer of restorative material, usually porcelain, is fitted onto the tooth surface, either to improve appearance or to protect a damaged tooth. Veneers are custom-designed and can cover worn enamel, uneven tooth alignment, crooked teeth and gaps. They can even widen smiles.

A thin layer of enamel is filed from the front of the teeth and the veneers are glued in place. Aged teeth are more likely to have chips, cracks or a generally worn, uneven appearance. Spaces in between can also get wider with the years and veneers can disguise these ageing signs as well as improving overall aesthetics, adding bulk to the teeth and plumping out the face.

Veneers can last up to fifteen years; after that replacements can be fitted. However, this is an irreversible process and is also expensive. Some dentists argue that it is an invasive procedure that may actually weaken teeth.

COST: FROM £500.

CROWNS

Crowns can be used to replace a large filling where there is not enough tooth left to hold the filling in place. They can also protect and restore weak, fractured teeth or poorly shaped teeth. They can be attached to dental bridges to replace missing teeth or to a dental implant. They are most commonly made from porcelain, metal or a combination of both, although porcelain crowns obviously give the most natural appearance.

COST: FROM £450.

EXPERT ADVICE FOR YOUTHFUL TEETH

How Not to Get Old asked Adam Slade of United Smile Centres for his top five anti-ageing tips for teeth.

1 GOOD DAILY MAINTENANCE is essential – including thorough brushing twice daily with a fluoride toothpaste and flossing.

2 DON'T SMOKE - it causes so many problems and nothing is worse for oral health.

3 AVOID foods and drinks that stain teeth.

4 VISIT A DENTAL HYGIENIST regularly.

5 AND LAST, but definitely not least, make sure you have regular check-ups with your dentist.

SAHRAE'S STORY (PART TWO)

Sahrae lost her front teeth in a bumper car accident when she was fifteen. Since then, she feels the missing teeth have affected her whole face, causing her to look older than her forty-four years. The problem has been made worse in the last three years due to some disappointing dental work which has left her with ill-fitting dentures and a hefty bill.

Because of the loss of her teeth and related soft tissue and bone shrinkage,

Sahrae's mouth area had lost its shape and no longer supported her lips and cheeks sufficiently. The severe wear to her remaining teeth and the missing support from her absent back teeth have caused her bite to over close. This has caused more wrinkles around her mouth and neck, and is also partly responsible for the loss of visible lip line. She would simply like to look her real age and feel attractive again.

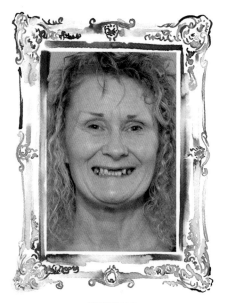

BEFORE

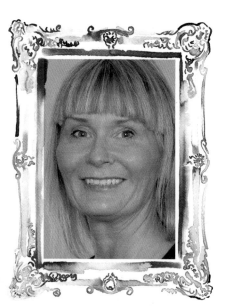

AFTER

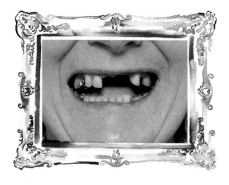

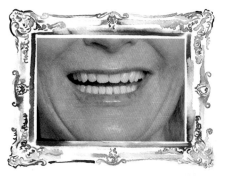

EXPERT PROFILES
DR CARL MANHEM, DR ADAM E SLADE AND MR JAMIE WRIGHT,
UNITED SMILE CENTRES

United Smile Centres specialize in implant and cosmetic restorative dentistry. Having met several different dentists offering a range of procedures, Sahrae was convinced she would get the right treatment for her from the team approach offered there.

United Smile Centres are the offspring of Chrysalis Dental Centres in Canada and United Smiles USA. The same protocols and techniques that have successfully treated thousands of North American patients with this same-day treatment are now being offered at USC London.

Dr Manhem carried out the surgical aspect of the upper jaw treatment and Dr Slade was responsible for the restoration of the lower jaw. Mr Wright worked with the surgeons to design and fabricate all the prosthetic teeth that will be utilized.

Dr Manhem qualified at the University of Gothenburg and at Dental College, University of Gothenburg in 1983. He completed his specialization in Oral Surgery in 1994 at the University of Linköping, Sweden and then worked as Assistant Professor at two university hospitals in the departments of Oral and Maxillofacial Surgery in Stockholm and then in Aarhus, Denmark. During this time he also worked at several implant clinics as well as a private hospital as a consultant, providing implant treatments to patients with all kinds of complex requirements.

Carl moved to the UK in 1998 and since then has been working at the Eastman Dental Institute, University College London, teaching implantology to postgraduate students. He is also involved in research on implants concerning healing processes and the biocompatibility of different implant materials. His clinical interests are implantology and reconstructive surgery.

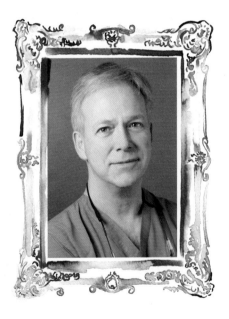

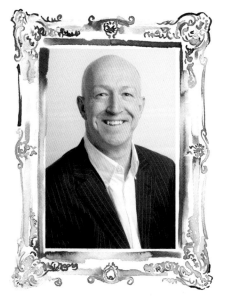

Dr Adam Slade qualified at Guy's Hospital, London in 1986 and after a few years in general dental practice he has focused on prosthodontics and implantology. He was awarded Master of Clinical Dentistry, Prosthodontics from London University in 2004. He is now involved in teaching a postgraduate programme to dentists worldwide and has a particular interest in cosmetic dentistry and advanced restorative care.

Jamie Wright is a clinical dental technician with more than twenty-five years' experience in dental technology. In 2004 he graduated from the International Denturist Education Centre and, in 2007, was one of the first to gain a diploma in Clinical Dental Technology from the Royal College of Surgeons. Jamie has worked with implant surgeons across the country, dedicating his care and attention to ensure a superior level of craftsmanship. His commitment to patient-focused treatment gained Jamie the Myerson International Best Aesthetic Award.

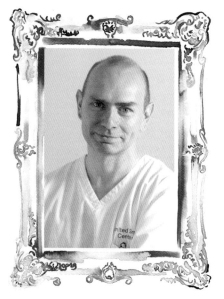

THE TREATMENT

From a dentist's point of view, Sahrae's case was an interesting one as it involved the whole spectrum of cosmetic dentistry. She had just six teeth remaining in the top arch. She was provided with several different treatment approaches before she elected to have them removed as they had been damaged by the previous dental work. This widened the options aesthetically. The condition of Sahrae's lower teeth was far better and it was decided to restore them. It was agreed to replace old fillings, create bridges and crowns where necessary, place a single dental implant and finally finish with very thin, porcelain veneers for the front bottom teeth to improve their general appearance.

After a long consultation it was agreed to place dental implants and immediately provide a new set of fixed teeth. Traditionally dental implants were placed under the gum and a three-month healing period was required before the teeth could be attached. During this period patients had to wear transitional dentures that were not attached to the implant and which, as a result, were cumbersome and inconvenient.

Recent technological advancement, however, has seen newer generations of dental implants with a treated surface and improved thread designs. This means that the implants used are much more stable on the day of fitting and, in the case of full arches of teeth, implants are rigidly joined together for even greater stability. As a result of this advancement it was now possible for the implants to support Sahrae's new upper teeth on the same day.

The benefits to Sahrae are enormous; because her new teeth are not supported on the gum, but by the bone below, there was less discomfort from the tooth extraction and healing was faster. Cumbersome transitional teeth were not required and Sahrae was able to leave the surgery on the same day with new fixed teeth that were used immediately. Furthermore, the approach used by the United Smile Centres team enables implants to be inserted in such a way that there is rarely any need for bone grafting, which is quite common with more traditional approaches.

Sahrae will return in four months for a titanium-reinforced definitive set of custom-made upper teeth to be fitted.

RECOVERY

Many patients experience remarkably little pain or swelling with this technique. However, it is still a surgical intervention and one can expect an initial recovery period of around two to four days. For the first few weeks following the procedure a slightly modified diet of softer food such as fish and pasta is suggested.

CARE OF IMPLANTS

Dental implants can preserve the structure of the jawbone, provide comfortable suport and retention for replacement teeth and restore facial aesthetics. Done well, the results can be truly amazing. It is important that implants are followed up and maintained at regular intervals to ensure their long-term health.

Sahrae will have check-ups at regular intervals for the first year and then a follow-up programme specific to her particular case will be recommended after that.

HAIR

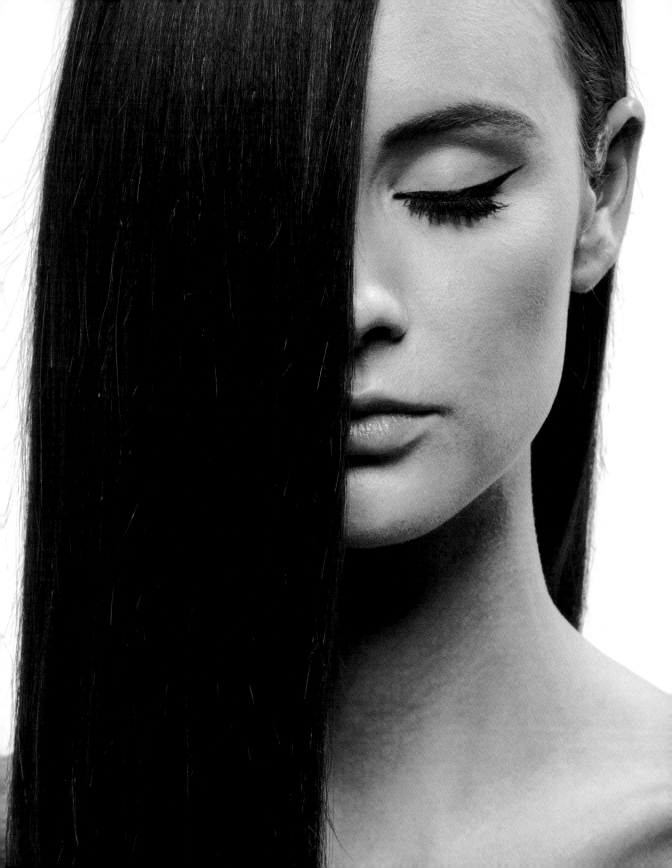

HOW THE DECADES
AFFECT YOUR HAIR

YOUR TWENTIES

◎ You are born with around 1,100 hair follicles for each square centimetre of scalp and no more follicles develop after birth.

◎ For most people the number of follicles will have fallen to 600 per square centimetre by the time they are in their twenties.

◎ Hair grows fastest between the ages of sixteen and twenty-four.

◎ Hair is the thickest it will ever be when you are twenty.

◎ Oil glands work overtime and hair quickly becomes greasy if it is not washed frequently.

◎ Light hair often starts to get darker.

◎ Some 20 per cent of men in their twenties notice their hair beginning to thin.

YOUR THIRTIES

◎ Male pattern baldness affects 30 per cent of thirty-year-olds.

◎ The first grey hairs appear.

◎ Very few people are natural blondes after the age of thirty.

◎ Hair becomes finer.

◎ Hair is more prone to damage and needs extra protection as less oil is produced.

HOW
NOT
TO
GET
OLD
102
HAIR

YOUR FORTIES

◎ The number of grey hairs multiplies because the body produces less melanin and pigment fades.

◎ The texture of hair changes, with grey hairs usually coarser and more wiry.

◎ For women, lower oestrogen levels mean thinner, drier hair.

YOUR FIFTIES

◎ About 50 per cent of men in their fifties are affected by male pattern baldness.

◎ Women's hair is also thinner as the menopause and loss of oestrogen take effect.

◎ Hormone fluctuations mean the loss of hair on your head can be accompanied by increased hair growth on the face.

◎ Some follicles produce only very fine, non-pigmented hairs.

YOUR SIXTIES

◎ Roughly 65 per cent of men are balding by the age of sixty.

◎ But the good news is that if you've reached sixty with no obvious signs of hair loss, the likelihood is you'll avoid it altogether – apart from the normal thinning that comes with age for both men and women.

◎ Grey hair usually turns white as pigment is lost.

◎ Oil gland production slows down, making hair much drier.

◎ Hair growth will have slowed to around 0.32 mm a day.

HOW
NOT
TO
GET
OLD
103
HAIR

HAIR ANATOMY

◎ HAIR IS COMPOSED OF 97 per cent protein. The other 3 per cent is made up of amino acids, minerals and trace elements (including silica).

◎ THE HAIR FOLLICLE is the cavity of cells embedded in the scalp at the base of the hair shaft, almost like a bulb.

◎ THE FOLLICLE is fed by a network of blood vessels that supply the nutrients needed for the hair to grow.

◎ THERE ARE NO NERVE CONNECTIONS to the hair, which is why it has no sensation or feeling.

◎ HAIR NORMALLY GROWS just over a centimetre a month but growth slows with age.

◎ WOMEN'S HAIR GROWS SLIGHTLY FASTER than men's – an extra 0.02 mm per day.

BLONDES HAVE MORE HAIR
The average human head has 100,000 hair follicles, each of which produces twenty individual hairs, but there are variations. Blondes have the highest number at 140,000 hair follicles; people with black hair tend to have around 110,000; brunettes match the average at 100,000; while redheads have the lowest number of follicles, with around 90,000.

HOW
NOT
TO
GET
OLD
**104
HAIR**

THE LIFE CYCLE OF A HAIR FOLLICLE

◎ **RESTING OR TELOGEN PHASE**

Between 10 and 15 per cent of your follicles will be in their resting phase at any one time.

◎ **TRANSITIONAL OR CATAGEN PHASE**

Following the resting phase, the follicle sheds its hair and grows a new one. This usually takes about three weeks.

◎ **GROWING OR ANAGEN PHASE**

The hair grows for between two and six years, after which the follicle goes into the resting phase again.

A healthy hair follicle continually repeats these three phases and individual follicles will be in different phases at any one time.

DID YOU KNOW?

STUDIES OF HUMAN BEHAVIOUR HAVE FOUND THAT 90 PER CENT OF MEN AND WOMEN WILL TOUCH THEIR HAIR WHEN AN ATTRACTIVE MEMBER OF THE OPPOSITE SEX WALKS TOWARDS THEM.

EAT YOUR WAY TO HEALTHY, YOUTHFUL HAIR

What you eat really affects the health of your hair. If you want lustrous, glossy, thick locks a balanced diet is always best. In particular, choose foods that are rich in the following nutrients.

HOW
NOT
TO
GET
OLD
**106
HAIR**

PROTEIN Found in oily fish, poultry, lean red meat, eggs and pulses.

OMEGA-3 FATTY ACIDS Found in oily fish, nuts such as walnuts and almonds, seeds including pumpkin and flax, avocados and leafy green vegetables.

OMEGA-9 Found in olives and olive oil, avocados and nuts.

VITAMINS Particularly B (eggs, wholegrains, beetroot), C (fresh fruit and vegetables), E (avocados, nuts, wholegrains).

MINERALS Zinc (oysters, crab, egg yolks, mushrooms), silica (oats, onions, wholewheat, beetroot), sulphur (broccoli and leafy green vegetables), magnesium (bananas, dried fruit, nuts).

BETA CAROTENE Orange, yellow and green fruits and vegetables.

IRON Dark chocolate, lean red meat, oily fish, leafy green vegetables. Anaemia, an acute lack of iron, can lead to hair loss.

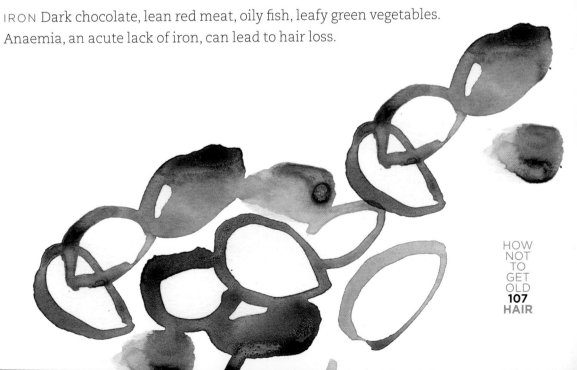

HOW
NOT
TO
GET
OLD
107
HAIR

TROUBLESHOOTING

◎ DRY, BRITTLE, lifeless hair can be a sign that you need to eat more essential fatty acids.

◎ OILY HAIR can be linked to a Vitamin B deficiency.

◎ DANDRUFF is often triggered by stress – the oil-producing glands can start to overwork causing dead cells to flake away in clumps.

◎ SLOW HAIR GROWTH or loss of colour may mean zinc is lacking from your diet.

◎ DRINKING too much alcohol robs your body of B Vitamins and can accelerate hair greying.

◎ AVOID EXTREME DIETS – they are a shock to the system and deprive your hair as well as your body of its basic nutritional needs.

DID YOU KNOW?

HAIR GROWS MORE SLOWLY IN COLD WEATHER WHEN CIRCULATION IS GENERALLY MORE SLUGGISH. YOU ALSO LOSE MORE HAIR IN SPRING AND AUTUMN AS YOUR BODY RESPONDS TO CHANGES IN THE SEASONS AND THE AMOUNT OF DAYLIGHT. SCIENTISTS HAVE DISCOVERED THAT PEOPLE SHED MORE HAIR IN NOVEMBER THAN IN ANY OTHER MONTH OF THE YEAR.

HAIR LOSS

Hair naturally thins as part of the ageing process. While the average twenty-year-old will have around 600 hairs per square centimetre, an average fifty-year-old will have less than 300. It is quite normal to shed between 100 and 125 hairs each day but these will be replaced. Hair loss happens when more than that number of hairs are lost and an increasing number of follicles shrink, resulting in a shorter growing phase, meaning shorter, thinner hairs and much more frequent shedding. Eventually the follicle stops producing hairs altogether and dies.

HOW
NOT
TO
GET
OLD
109
HAIR

FEMALE HAIR LOSS

Women's hair naturally thins with age but this is usually less noticeable than male hair loss because it decreases evenly across the whole scalp rather than in distinct bald patches. However, around 30 per cent of women will have a problem with thinning hair at some point in their life, and because hair is so linked to ideas of femininity, this can have a particularly damaging psychological impact on women. Female hair loss can be down to genetic factors but the reasons are usually much more varied and, as a result, can be trickier to both diagnose and treat.

Women who think they may have a problem should always seek medical advice and see their doctor for a complete check-up and blood tests to identify any underlying conditions.

The most common causes of female hair loss include:

◎ PREGNANCY Normal daily hair loss stops during pregnancy so that by the end of the pregnancy hair looks particularly thick and glossy. The flip side to this is that hair is shed rapidly after childbirth and takes a few months to settle down.

◎ HORMONAL CHANGES, including stopping birth control pills. This is nearly always temporary.

◎ POOR DIET, including sudden changes in diet or crash dieting. A lack of iron, Vitamins B and C and essential fatty acids and minerals can all contribute to hair thinning and loss.

◎ STRESS OR TRAUMA Both emotional stress and anxiety and trauma after a physical accident or surgery can cause hair problems. Try a gentle scalp massage to soothe your emotions and stimulate the hair follicles.

◎ SOME PRESCRIPTION MEDICATIONS have been linked to hair loss – ask your doctor for advice. Vitamin A derivatives, including Tretinoin, which is prescribed for some skin conditions, can lead to hypervitaminosis A and cause hair to thin.

◎ MORE SERIOUS GYNAECOLOGICAL conditions, thyroid disease and medication and lupus can also be underlying causes. Medical diagnosis and treatment will be necessary.

HOW
NOT
TO
GET
OLD
110
HAIR

AS WELL AS MAKING HAIR LOOK FULLER
AND MORE LUSTROUS, PREGNANCY CAN ALSO
CHANGE THE TEXTURE AND COLOUR,
EVEN MAKING HAIR CURLIER.

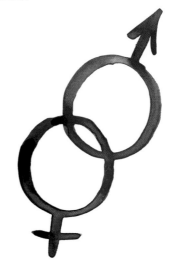

MALE HAIR LOSS

Male pattern baldness is largely genetically programmed and can be inherited from either the mother or the father. The most common form is called androgenetic alopecia and is triggered when falling levels of the hormone testosterone are converted to dihydrotestosterone (DHT), which attacks hair follicles causing them to shrink and ultimately stop producing hairs. Certain areas of the head have more of the enzyme that makes DHT in the cells around the hair shaft, which is why there is a pattern to hair thinning and loss.

HOW
NOT
TO
GET
OLD
111
HAIR

NON-SURGICAL TREATMENTS

FINASTERIDE

Also known as Propecia®, finasteride was approved by the US Food and Drug Administration in 1997 but is only suitable for men. It works by blocking one of the enzymes that convert testosterone into DHT. Clinical trials show that with continued use it helps to preserve existing hair for many men and will actually increase hair growth for some.

Side effects can include allergic reactions, headaches, impotence and loss of libido, though these are often temporary and figures suggest just a small percentage of men are affected.

MINOXIDIL®

Minoxidil is a topical, clear liquid or foam which is applied directly to the scalp. It is thought to work by increasing blood flow to the scalp and hair follicles, increasing the supply of nutrients which encourages hair to grow. This can be used by women as well as men who can also use Minoxidil+Progesterone. While not a cure for baldness, it can slow hair loss, help to retain existing hair and promote hair growth. Results usually show after four months.

Side effects are minimal but include headaches, rashes and mild facial hair growth.

HOW
NOT
TO
GET
OLD
112
HAIR

LASER HAIR THERAPY

Using red light or phototherapy
(in the form of a laser comb or cap,
or a clinic-based laser), the low-level
energy delivered to the scalp is thought
to reduce swelling around the follicle
that is being choked by DHT. It increases
blood flow and nutrients to stimulate
hair growth. Regular treatments over
a period of three to five months can
result in thicker healthier hair.

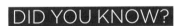

DID YOU KNOW?

SOME FORM OF HAIR LOSS
AFFECTS OVER 30 MILLION MEN AND
20 MILLION WOMEN IN THE US.

HAIR TRANSPLANTS

Modern hair transplant techniques really date from the 1930s in Japan where they were only used for eyebrows or eyelashes. Transplants to treat baldness began in the late 1950s in New York. Since then, techniques have advanced, offering far more successful, natural-looking results.

Hair transplants do not work for everyone. Follicles for the transplant are harvested from an area of permanent hairs which are unaffected by conditions such as male pattern baldness. This donor area is typically at the back or sides of the head. Everyone has a finite amount of permanent donor hair and so care must be taken to make best use of this limited supply. Some patients achieve the desired effect with a single surgical procedure, but most will need more than one to increase hair density or treat ongoing hair loss.

Women as well as men have benefited from hair transplants but because the causes of hair thinning for women are more wide-ranging, only around a third of women would be suitable candidates.

HOW
NOT
TO
GET
OLD
114
HAIR

FOLLICULAR UNIT EXTRACTION (FUE)

This is the technique of extracting individual follicular units from the donor area, leaving only 'dot' scars which allow the hair to be worn even shorter than a Strip procedure would allow. It is more time-consuming and the yield of donor hairs is not as high as the Strip method. The hair at the back and sides of the head needs to be shaved to a couple of mm in order to perform FUE. The follicular units can be extracted by hand or with robotic assistance. Once extracted, the follicular unit grafts are transplanted in the same way as those from a Strip procedure.

FOLLICULAR UNIT TRANSPLANTATION (FUT)

Also known as the Strip procedure, so called because a thin strip of donor hair is harvested from an area of the patient's permanent hair. The strip is removed under local anaesthetic and the area, which is usually at the back of the head, is sutured. The width of the scar varies from patient to patient but it is instantly concealed by hair worn at grade 4 (12 mm) or longer. This method allows a surgeon to harvest the maximum possible number of grafts in a patient's lifetime.

Once the strip is harvested it is dissected into microscopic grafts of individual follicular units with between one and four hairs in each. These grafts are then kept in cold tissue storage until they are implanted into balding areas of the scalp. It takes a skilled surgeon to place the grafts to ensure the hair looks natural and gives the impression of the most hair. Usually one-hair grafts are placed at the front of the hairline, two-hair grafts immediately behind and the three- and four-hair units in the central area.

HOW
NOT
TO
GET
OLD
**115
HAIR**

RECOVERY

After the surgery, small scabs and redness develop on the implant sites, which begin to fall off naturally during the first week. They should not be scratched as this could cause infection or dislodge the graft. On the sixth post-operative day the grafts are secure and can be touched and washed normally.

Patients are usually prescribed pain and anti-swelling medication and may be prescribed antibiotics. Many patients find that they do not require painkillers after a couple of days. Vitamin E and anti-inflammatories should be avoided for a week after the procedure. Alcohol and smoking are also off-limits since they impair healing and can affect the blood and blood pressure. Exercise and strenuous activity should be avoided for ten days. Most people take a week off work.

Like any surgical procedure, there can be swelling, bruising and some redness. It's not unusual for the forehead to swell, especially if most of the implants were towards the hairline and front of the head. Swelling typically peaks on the third day but is usually gone by the end of a week. Forehead massage and ice packs can help. There is sometimes a degree of numbness in the donor and transplant areas, which can last over a year but usually disappears after a few weeks.

If stitches have been used, they are removed ten to fourteen days after surgery.

RESULTS

Implanted hair takes time to develop its own blood supply but will then grow as normal. Follicles often go into a resting phase immediately after transplant and may shed their hair two to four weeks afterwards. Hair growth usually starts after three months with the bulk of the change between five and ten months, though it can take longer.

COST: DEPENDS ON THE NUMBER OF GRAFTS TRANSPLANTED BUT AN AVERAGE-SIZED HAIR TRANSPLANT COSTS ANYTHING FROM £3,500 TO £5,000.

HOW
NOT
TO
GET
OLD
116
HAIR

CALLUM'S STORY

Callum first noticed his hairline receding when he was just eighteen years old. It's a myth that male pattern baldness is inherited only from the maternal line – both Callum's father and grandfather also lost their hair at an early age.

Now twenty-seven, Callum feels that his hair loss is making him look older and it is badly affecting his confidence. He has previously thought about taking medication to combat the problem but has always been concerned about possible side effects.

Callum was consulted by Mr Edward Ball, hair transplant surgeon at Ziering's London clinic. Mr Ball explained the importance of considering medication to control his ongoing hair loss: an important issue in view of his finite donor supply and relatively young age. Callum opted to take the Propecia® tablets and topical Minoxidil foam in an attempt to halt his hair loss and hopefully thicken the other areas of hair that have started to thin.

They discussed the various methods for hair transplantation, including Follicular Unit Extraction (FUE), using the latest robotic ARTAS® System offered by Ziering. The Ziering Robograft™ technique uses the ARTAS System to harvest consistently high-quality grafts without leaving the line scar from the more traditional Follicula Unit Transplantation (FUT) or Strip method. However, Callum never intends to wear his hair so short that a line scar would be a problem and decided on the FUT/Strip method which will provide a greater yield of donor hair in his lifetime. He is aware that he is likely to require more surgery in the future to add density to his new area of growth or address some areas of ongoing hair loss.

Callum was a little anxious about possible pain during the procedure but was pleasantly surprised that he could hardly feel the anaesthetic injections and went on to feel nothing while his transplant was carried out. Half an hour or so was spent lying face down while the Strip was extracted and stitched. He then watched DVDs while the team of hair technician dissected the Strip under microscopes to produce follicular unit grafts in their naturally occurring groupings of 1, 2, 3 or 4 hairs. Meanwhile Mr Ball made the 2,221 incisions which would determine the design and distribution of the transplanted hair. Finally the grafts were painstakingly inserted, one by one, into these incisions in a pattern which would reproduce a natural-looking hairline and frontal third of his scalp. When the last of the grafts had been inserted, Callum was able to take a look in the mirror and get an idea of the impact his new hairline would give him.

After a long day or surgery Callum was tired but excited about his new head of hair. Next comes the difficult wait for the growth of his new hair and boost in his self-confidence.

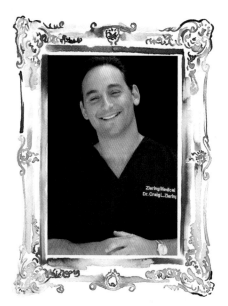

EXPERT PROFILE
DR CRAIG ZIERING

Dr Ziering is the Founder and Medical Director of Ziering, which specializes exclusively in hair restoration. Based in the US, his role involves leading his team of hair transplant surgeons and introducing industry-leading standards in medical care and patient satisfaction.

He received his Doctorate of Osteopathic Medicine from Nova Southeastern University in Miami, Florida, and completed his residency at Ohio University's Grandview Medical Centre in Dayton, Ohio. He is now a well-respected and extremely popular hair transplant surgeon, having completed over 18,000 procedures in his more than twenty-year career. He has developed his own surgical techniques and technology to achieve extraordinary results. Consistently at the forefront of the latest advances, he is a pioneer in the field of robotic hair restoration and remains passionate about his patients and this evolving field of medicine.

Dr Ziering is a registered member of the International and European Societies of Hair Restoration Surgery, the American Board of Hair Restoration Surgery, the American Osteopathic College and Academy of Dermatology, the American Society of Dermatologic Surgery, and the American Academy of Anti-Ageing Medicine. An ISHRS Faculty Lecturer, Dr. Ziering was recently selected to be Chairman of the Medical Advisory Board for Biologix and to serve on the Hair Foundation Scientific Advisory Council as well as continuing his work as the Primary Investigator for Histogen.

HOW
NOT
TO
GET
OLD
118
HAIR

EXPERT PROFILE
MR EDWARD BALL

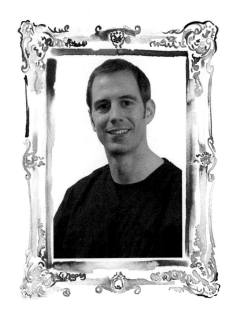

Mr Edward Ball is a hair transplant surgeon and the Clinical Director of Ziering UK. A member of the Royal College of Surgeons of England, Mr Ball draws on his years of experience in hair restoration, plastic surgery, dermatology, general practice and aesthetic medicine to provide patients with a holistic, first-class service.

Mr Ball is continually looking to improve upon established techniques and embrace new technology so that his patients consistently receive world-class results. He trained in hair restoration in the US, having been handpicked to undertake his Fellowship in Hair Restoration Surgery with Dr Craig Ziering of Beverly Hills. In February 2013, he was the first surgeon to offer robot-assisted Follicular Unit Extraction with the ARTAS System to patients in the United Kingdom at Ziering's London clinic. Mr Ball had been one of Dr Ziering's first patients in California to undergo a procedure using the ARTAS System and his ability to empathize with his patients has been greatly enhanced by this experience.

Trained in microsurgery, Mr Ball is a valued member of the skin cancer surgery team at University Hospital Southampton and serves on the Medical Advisory Board for Biologix Hair Inc. He is an active member of the International Society of Hair Restoration Surgery, the British Society of Hair Restoration Surgery, Royal College of General Practitioners, and the British College of Aesthetic Medicine. Mr Ball is also a teacher and mentor to novice surgeons new to the field and has been published in highly respected medical journals such as *The British Journal of Plastic Surgery*, *The British Journal of Dermatology*, *The Journal of Plastic and Reconstructive Surgery*, *Burns Journal* and *Clinical and Experimental Dermatology*.

HOW
NOT
TO
GET
OLD
119
HAIR

EXPERT
ADVICE FOR HEALTHY HAIR

'When it comes to having healthy hair, it's not only what you apply to it but how you look after yourself holistically, too', says Dr Ziering.

The effects of stress, lack of sleep and a poor diet may show themselves on your skin first, but over time they affect your hair just as obviously.

◎ EAT A HEALTHY DIET, including plenty of protein.

◎ OMEGA-3 essential fatty acids help to keep hair and scalp healthy and hydrated.

◎ LEAFY GREEN VEGETABLES provide vital vitamins and minerals.

◎ DRINK WATER – important for keeping you and your hair hydrated.

◎ AVOID SMOKING.

◎ CONTROL YOUR STRESS LEVELS – easier said than done but stress can interfere with hair growth.

◎ SORT OUT any hormonal imbalances – hormones affect hair growth.

◎ A GOOD NIGHT'S SLEEP helps to restore balance throughout the body.

HOW
NOT
TO
GET
OLD
**120
HAIR**

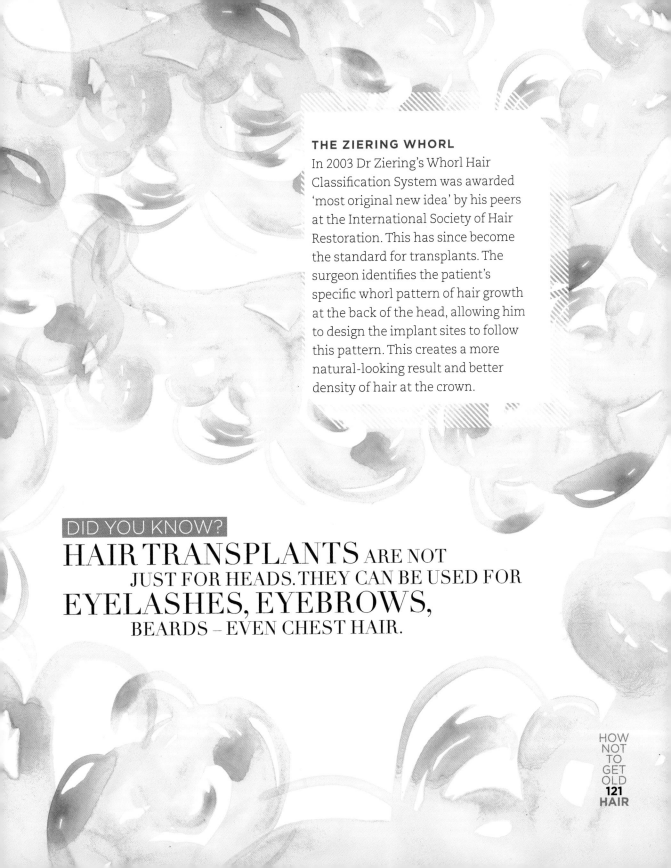

THE ZIERING WHORL

In 2003 Dr Ziering's Whorl Hair Classification System was awarded 'most original new idea' by his peers at the International Society of Hair Restoration. This has since become the standard for transplants. The surgeon identifies the patient's specific whorl pattern of hair growth at the back of the head, allowing him to design the implant sites to follow this pattern. This creates a more natural-looking result and better density of hair at the crown.

DID YOU KNOW?

HAIR TRANSPLANTS ARE NOT JUST FOR HEADS. THEY CAN BE USED FOR EYELASHES, EYEBROWS, BEARDS – EVEN CHEST HAIR.

HOW
NOT
TO
GET
OLD
**121
HAIR**

SURGICAL TOP TEN

The following tables show the UK's most popular surgical procedures in 2012, based on the number of procedures carried out.

WOMEN AND MEN

1	Breast augmentation	9,854	↓ 1.6 per cent
2	Blepharoplasty (eyelid surgery)	6,829	↑ 12.7 per cent
3	Face/neck lift	5,660	↑ 14 per cent
4	Breast reduction	4,859	↓ 8.2 per cent
5	Rhinoplasty	4,180	↓ 7.5 per cent
6	Liposuction	3,071	↓ 14.2 per cent
7	Abdominoplasty	2,989	↓ 11.5 per cent
8	Fat transfer	2,882	↑ 13 per cent
9	Brow lift	1,812	↑ 17 per cent
10	Otoplasty (ear correction)	1,066	↑ 8.9 per cent

There were 43,172 procedures in total carried out on women and men in 2012, an increase of 0.2 per cent on the previous year.

HOW
NOT
TO
GET
OLD
122
**SURGICAL
TOP TEN**

WOMEN ONLY

1	Breast augmentation	9,843	↓ 1.6 per cent
2	Blepharoplasty (eyelid surgery)	6,070	↑ 13 per cent
3	Face/neck lift	5,324	↑ 13.3 per cent
4	Breast reduction	4,217	↓ 6.3 per cent
5	Rhinoplasty	3,228	↓ 7 per cent
6	Abdominoplasty	2,882	↓ 11 per cent
7	Fat transfer	2,641	↑ 13 per cent
8	Liposuction	2,638	↓ 14 per cent
9	Brow lift	1,663	↑ 17 per cent
10	Otoplasty (ear correction)	563	↓ 13 per cent

Women had 39,070 procedures in 2012 and accounted for 90.5 per cent of all cosmetic procedures. This was an increase of 0.8 per cent on 2011.

MEN ONLY

1	Rhinoplasty	952	↓ 9 per cent
2	Blepharoplasty (eyelid surgery)	758	↑ 11 per cent
3	Breast reduction	642	↓ 18 per cent
4	Otoplasty (ear correction)	503	↓ 3.5 per cent
5	Liposuction	433	↓ 15 per cent
6	Face/neck lift	306	↓ 14 per cent
7	Fat transfer	241	↑ 9.5 per cent
8	Brow lift	149	↑ 19 per cent
9	Abdominoplasty	107	↓ 14 per cent
10	Breast augmentation	11	no change

Overall the 4,102 procedures carried out saw a fall of 4.5 per cent on 2011 but there were increases in the figures for anti-ageing surgeries for men.

(All figures from BAAPS, 28.1.2013)

HOW
NOT
TO
GET
OLD
123
SURGICAL
TOP TEN

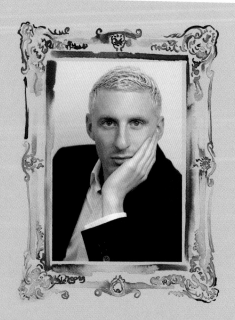

MORE THAN SKIN DEEP

BY DR MAX PEMBERTON

It's only human to want a quick fix to the problems we have in life. Plastic surgery and anti-ageing procedures are appealing because they offer quick, easy and sometimes even instantaneous results. What's not to love? Well, sometimes the change we're really looking for is not going to be achieved by surgery. As a doctor working in mental health, I do worry that, for some people, the motivation behind changing their appearance is more than just cosmetic. There could be an underlying, more emotional, problem that leads them to want to change how they look.

HOW
NOT
TO
GET
OLD
124
**MORE THAN
SKIN DEEP**

I should say from the outset that I have nothing against people going under the knife if that's what they choose to do and they have realistic expectations about what they want it to achieve. What I would always advise, though, is that you think carefully – not just about the procedure you're thinking of having, but about what you hope it will do for you and how you think it will change your life.

Any good surgeon will tell you that they often see people in their clinics who are really there because of family, relationship or emotional difficulties that no operation or injection can ever hope of correcting. If you're having relationship problems, for example, having a breast enlargement might make you feel more confident with your husband and he might even pay you more attention, but it's not going to fundamentally change the nature of your relationship. It's an uncomfortable truth, but sometimes, it's what's going on in your relationship that you need to change, not your appearance.

Of course, much is made of the physical risks associated with cosmetic surgery, but less attention is paid to the psychological risks. People usually assume that, if you're unhappy with a particular part of your body or appearance, then getting it fixed can only be a good thing. In fact, research has shown it's not quite that simple.

Studies have shown that, for those with underlying emotional or psychological problems, such as depression, undergoing plastic surgery can sometimes make patients feel worse. The reason for this is that they place a great deal of importance on the surgery as a way of making them feel better about themselves and if it doesn't, they can feel hopeless. Actually, in some cases, their appearance may not be the root cause of their unhappiness and the desire for surgery just a manifestation of deeper problems that would be better addressed through talking therapies.

HOW
NOT
TO
GET
OLD
125
**MORE THAN
SKIN DEEP**

It's true that sometimes correcting an imperfection can make us feel better about ourselves and more confident. This can have a positive impact on our careers, our relationships and our sex lives. But it would be wrong to think that it holds the answer to every problem in our lives, or even our overall sense of self worth. Studies have shown that people who undergo cosmetic surgery report afterwards that they find the part of their body that was operated on more attractive. But, on the whole, they do not report feeling more satisfied with their overall appearance. So people with cosmetic improvements might be happy with the results, but ultimately, might not rate their own mirror image any better than they used to.

I've often seen patients who have tried surgery and who, after the initial boost of self esteem following the operation, go back to being unhappy – not because the operation didn't work, but because it was never really their breasts, or their nose or wrinkles that were the problems. It was something more fundamental such as low self-esteem or a lack of self worth, perhaps with roots in childhood or adolescence, or because of past relationships. Often when someone needs to grapple with these kinds of problems, it's easier for them to focus on a part of their body that they don't think is quite right, rather than the actual issue. Interestingly, people who are considering surgery but who undergo talking therapy to address their low mood or feelings of low self esteem often decide afterwards that they feel they don't need the operation after all.

It's not unusual for those suffering from Body Dysmorphic Disorder (BDD) to look into cosmetic surgery. BDD is a condition whereby people fixate on one particular part of their body and wrongly think that there is a problem with it. A good surgeon should spot this and refer the patient to a psychiatrist, as they are suffering from a problem that

HOW
NOT
TO
GET
OLD
126
MORE THAN
SKIN DEEP

surgery won't really address. Research shows that for people with BDD, surgery can make them feel worse and that what will actually help will be talking therapy and, in some cases, medication.

If you are considering undergoing cosmetic surgery, think carefully about the real reasons you want to have it done. Go to at least two surgeons to get their opinion about what can be realistically achieved and listen to them if they suggest that, actually, your expectations are unlikely to be met.

If you're feeling low, depressed or have poor self-esteem or confidence, then you could consider having a short course of Cognitive Behavioural Therapy (CBT) before you make any decisions about surgery. Surgery will always be there as an option further down the line. There's no rush. You might save a lot of money and future disappointment by addressing any psychological problems first and then seeing if you still really feel you need surgery.

It's fine to change what you're dissatisfied with, but remember, life is not necessarily going to get better by simply having surgery.

HOW
NOT
TO
GET
OLD
127
**MORE THAN
SKIN DEEP**

THE
BODY

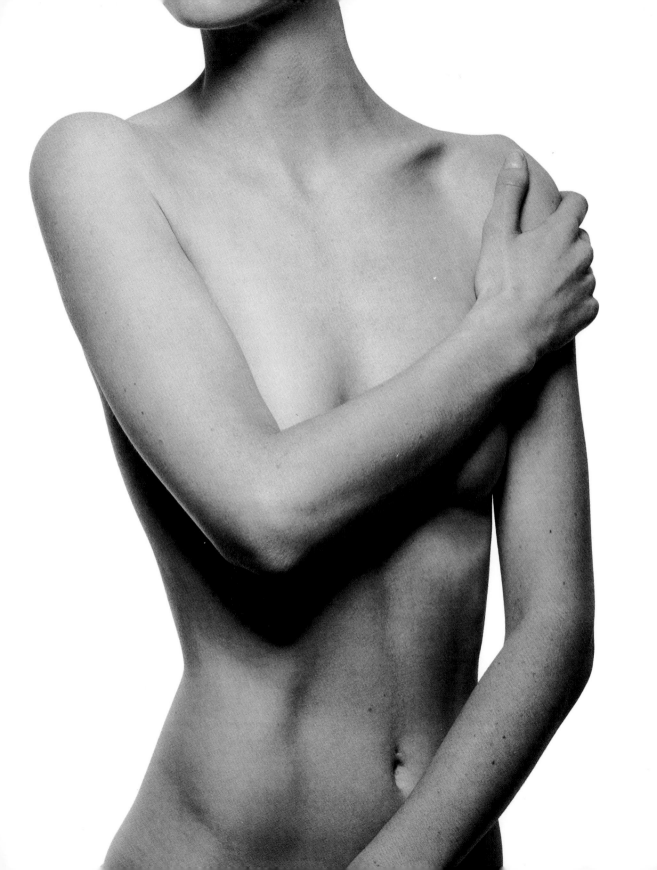

Many of the same factors that age the face are also responsible for body ageing but what's happening on the inside is probably even more important; while we are all keen to look young, it is vital to actually feel young. If you are healthy and energetic you are always going to create an impression of youth. What we do, the way we eat, the exercise we take, and how we look after ourselves all determine how well our bodies age.

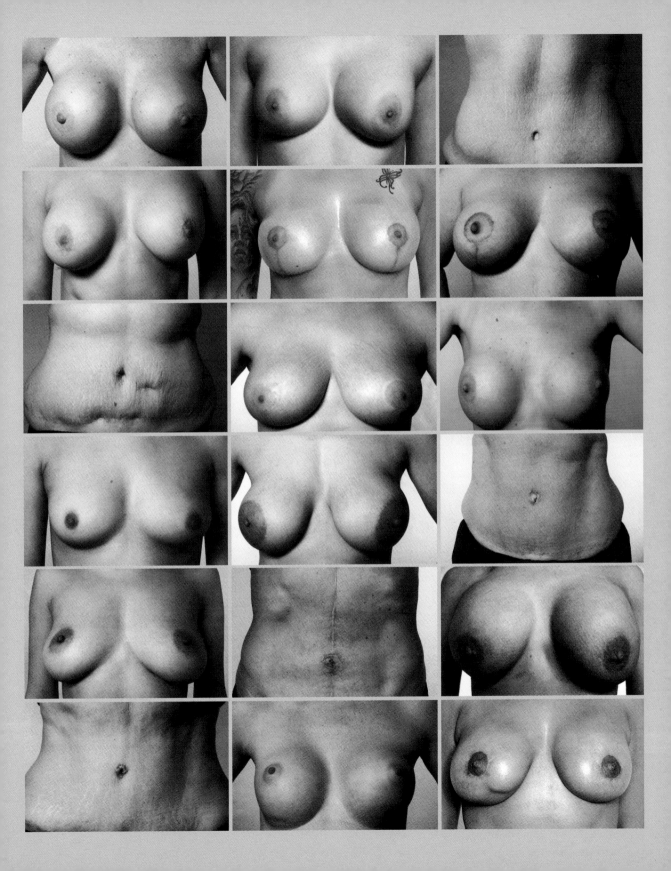

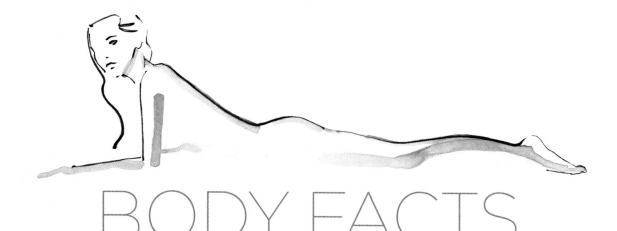

BODY FACTS

COLLAGEN not only gives skin its strength and elasticity, it is also the main component of all connective tissue, accounting for between 25 and 35 per cent of all the protein in the body. It is found mainly in fibrous tissues such as tendons and ligaments, and also in bone, muscle, cartilage, blood vessels, the gut and the discs in your spine.

WITH AGE, COLLAGEN PRODUCTION SLOWS, the cell structure weakens and is prone to mutation, ligaments and tendons become less flexible and joints stiffen. Free radical damage from the effects of the sun, smoking, pollution and diet accelerates this ageing process.

DEVELOPING GOOD HABITS early on can really help to slow the decline. Exercising and eating a healthy diet are a good place to start (see pages 168–215). And avoid yo-yo dieting – it puts a strain on your whole body and dramatic weight loss often leaves you with excess skin that no amount of exercise can tone or shift.

CARE FOR THE SKIN ON YOUR BODY as you would your face. It's very easy to neglect and just hide it away beneath layers of clothes. Remember it's your body's largest organ and needs nourishment from inside and out.

HOW
NOT
TO
GET
OLD
132
THE BODY

EATING ESSENTIAL FATTY ACIDS, antioxidant beta carotene and Vitamin E from oily fish, vegetables, nuts and seeds will help keep skin healthy, supple and fresh. And choose moisturizing body creams with the same anti-ageing antioxidant ingredients you look for in a face cream.

REGULAR EXFOLIATION is even more important to keep skin from looking dull and to slough away dead surface cells. Body brushing and gentle massage with a loofah or salt scrub can all help to boost circulation, supplying skin with nutrients and removing waste products. A short blast of cold water at the end of your shower also helps to wake up your skin.

ALWAYS USE SUN PROTECTION The skin on your neck, chest and breasts is just as delicate and often thinner than skin on your face and there are fewer oil glands to protect from wrinkles and pigmentation. Wear a minimum SPF 15 and don't forget the backs of your hands – a real giveaway when it comes to age.

STAND TALL Your posture makes such a difference to your appearance and overall confidence. Try to relax your shoulders; much of the tension we all carry round with us settles there, creating back and neck problems.

LASTLY, AND PERHAPS MOST IMPORTANTLY, DRINK WATER At least eight glasses of still water a day is recommended. Water is vital for life: it makes up roughly 70 per cent of your body and is involved in virtually every body process. If you're dehydrated, your skin will look older and more lined, your metabolism will be sluggish and your circulation will be slow. You'll lack energy and find it harder to concentrate. Apart from drinking it, remember that vegetables such as cucumber, and fruit including watermelon and grapefruit, are also good sources of water.

HOW
NOT
TO
GET
OLD
133
THE BODY

SURGICAL BODY TREATMENTS

There has never been a wider range of treatments available, aimed at correcting whatever imperfection you may feel age and life in general have thrown at you. The claims are impressive but the hype (and the cost) can far exceed the results and, if done badly, some of these 'cures' can cause serious, even permanent, damage.

Before opting for any treatment or surgery take time to do your research. Talk to several different clinics or practitioners before coming to a decision and always make sure you understand exactly what is involved, the sort of results you can realistically expect and the recovery time. Don't be nervous about asking to see before and after photographs, referrals, and case studies, and don't forget to find out about risks and possible side effects.

For more information on choosing an experienced, properly qualified surgeon and what qualifications to look out for, see pages 49–51. You can also find further details from the British Association of Plastic Surgery (BAPS), the British Association of Aesthetic Plastic Surgeons (BAAPS) and from the General Medical Council (see Directory, page 233).

HOW
NOT
TO
GET
OLD
134
THE BODY

PRE-SURGERY

It is important to make sure you are as healthy as possible before any operation, not only for your own safety during the surgery but also to help you make a good recovery afterwards and to ensure it is as successful as it can be.

If you are planning to lose weight, it is better to do so beforehand. You should give up smoking as this seriously affects healing, and stick to a balanced diet and exercise.

You will also be advised by your surgeon on anything you should specifically avoid in the weeks prior to the operation – this will include various prescription and other medications, multivitamins, Vitamin E, fish oils and anti-inflammatories.

The British Association of Aesthetic Plastic Surgeons (BAAPS) offers the following guidelines on cosmetic and plastic surgery:

◎ Make your own decisions.
◎ Be informed – remember, no surgery or procedure is 100 per cent risk free.
◎ Be comfortable – with the organization, surgeon and clinic.
◎ Know your surgeon. BAAPS can help you find a properly qualified and experienced surgeon in your area.
◎ Get the timing right. Surgery is traumatic enough – it should be avoided if you have recently had a major life event.
◎ Beware of 'free' consultations, likewise booking fees and non-returnable deposits.
◎ Think about location.
◎ Talk to your GP for an unbiased view from someone with your health and welfare in mind.
◎ You can always change your mind.
◎ Take your time – don't rush into surgery.
(from BAAPS consumer safety guidelines)

HOW
NOT
TO
GET
OLD
135
THE BODY

BREASTS

Breast size is largely genetically programmed but the ageing process can alter their youthful shape; gravity seems to take its toll as breasts shrink and begin to droop. The fibrous bands that support the breasts begin to break down and the skin stretches. Pregnancy, breastfeeding and weight fluctuations, especially dramatic weight loss, all add to the process.

HOW
NOT
TO
GET
OLD
136
THE BODY

BREAST AUGMENTATION

This has been the most common cosmetic procedure in the UK for many years and recovery is now much faster than it used to be. In the past, implants had to go behind the muscle, which was painful. Newer techniques mean fibres can be separated, allowing implants to be placed in front of the muscle and thereby speeding up recovery.

TYPES OF IMPLANT

Two types of implant are commonly used in the UK:

◎ SILICONE GEL IMPLANTS
These are available as a liquid, a gel, or a solid form similar to plastic.

◎ SALINE IMPLANTS
These are filled with sterile salt water.

Each type has associated advantages and disadvantages, although in practice, most are made from silicone. The recent enquiry into PIP implants concluded there was no significant risk to health, although as they are more likely to rupture, they are not recommended. With saline implants, it is sometimes possible to see the liquid moving under the skin.

SHAPE OF IMPLANT

The traditional shape is round but teardrop-shaped implants are now also available. The round shape can give more fullness in the upper half of the breast, which is often where women particularly want it. In practice the round implants tend to settle into something resembling a teardrop shape when in position. Round implants are more fluid and teardrops more rigid, which can cause a problem as implants can move around and rotate in the body pocket created for them. This shift would be very obvious with the teardrop shape.

COMPLICATIONS

Alongside normal surgical complications, the body can react to the implant. This happens in roughly 5 or 6 per cent of patients after a year or so. This can result in pain and a hardening of the implant. In extreme cases, the implant would need to be removed. Infection can also develop around an implant.

Breast size and shape takes time to settle and sometimes it may exaggerate any asymmetry between breasts. Larger breasts don't always result in a cleavage.

RECOVERY

Patients should sleep propped up for the first two weeks and are advised to wear an elastic support garment. They should avoid lifting or exercise for six weeks.

COST: FROM £4,000.

BREAST LIFT (MASTOPEXY)

Here, surgery reshapes the breast to look more youthful and feel firmer. Excess skin is removed from underneath each breast and the breast itself is tightened and the nipples repositioned at a higher level. The size of the areola can also be reduced at the same time.

SURGEONS use different techniques for uplifting breasts. A common method involves three incisions. One incision is made around the nipple area. Another runs vertically from the bottom edge of the areola to the crease beneath the breast. The third incision is made horizontally underneath the breast and follows the natural curve of the breast crease. After the plastic surgeon has removed excess breast skin, the nipple and areola are shifted to a higher position and if the areola has stretched due to sagging it will be reduced in size. Skin that was formerly located above the areola is brought down underneath it to reshape the breast.

IT IS ADVISABLE to wait until you have finished having children, as pregnancy is likely to stretch breasts again. If you also want to increase fullness, an uplift could be accompanied by implants, although this can increase the rate at which breasts begin to droop again.

COMPLICATIONS

Women can be left with some numbness to their nipples and may not be able to breastfeed afterwards. Scarring can be reduced with different techniques. There are the usual risks associated with general anaesthetics and surgery, and occasionally heavy bleeding or infection.

RECOVERY

As with augmentation, you should expect to take it easy for around six weeks and refrain from any lifting or exercise during that time. Support garments may be advised and patients should sleep propped up for the first couple of weeks.

COST: FROM £4,000.

HOW
NOT
TO
GET
OLD
138
THE BODY

BREAST REDUCTION (REDUCTION MAMMOPLASTY)

Reduction mammoplasty is used to reduce the size and change the shape of breasts. Excess fat and skin are removed from the breasts, which are then reshaped and the nipples repositioned to create smaller breasts. This can be used to correct asymmetry, where one breast is much bigger than the other. It should only be carried out after breasts have stopped growing, but pregnancy and weight loss or gain can alter the size again after the operation.

Traditional mammoplasty takes several hours under general anaesthetic. An alternative is now offered in the form of a Microlipo breast reduction, which claims to allow reduction without the need for major surgery. It is minimally invasive and so allows rapid post-operative recovery and a quick return to normal activities with minimal scarring.

SIDE EFFECTS
Nipples are likely to be less sensitive and there can be numbness. Few women will be able to breastfeed following surgery.

COMPLICATIONS
Risks are the same as for other breast operations. Sometimes a follow-up procedure with a local anaesthetic will be needed to adjust any folds of skin at the ends of scars.

RECOVERY
Slightly less time is needed than for an augmentation or uplift.

COST: £5,000+, BUT IS SOMETIMES AVAILABLE ON THE NHS.

MALE BREAST REDUCTION (GYNECOMASTIA)

Enlarged breasts on men, or man boobs (sometimes called 'moobs'), is quite a common problem. Occasionally caused by certain medications, drugs or some diseases, they are more often associated with age, affecting as many as one in three older men.

If the problem is largely due to excess fatty tissue this can be removed by liposuction. If excess glandular tissue is to blame this can only be removed surgically. Sometimes a combination of both is suggested. Most operations take around ninety minutes, usually under general anaesthetic, although sometimes local anaesthesia and sedation are used.

The surgeon will make an incision around the areola and liposuction may be used to suck out fatty tissue. Depending on the amount of tissue to be removed, cuts may extend down the chest from the areola and the nipples may need to be repositioned.

RECOVERY

It takes some time for the full effect to emerge. Initially there will be swelling and bruising and the patient should wear an elastic pressure garment for up to two weeks. Exercise or any strenuous activity should be avoided for about three weeks and it can take up to six weeks to fully return to normal activities. Occasionally results can be uneven and there may be a loss of sensation.

COST: FROM £2,000 BY LIPOSUCTION AND FROM £5,400 FOR AN EXCISION TECHNIQUE.

AUTOLOGOUS FAT TRANSFER TO THE BREAST – THE WAY FORWARD?

This is not new as such, in that fat transfer or lipofilling has been around for at least a hundred years. In the past it has always been problematic for breast augmentation, with fat cells dying and causing cysts or calcification which can show up on mammograms and, it was thought, mimic cancer.

However, new techniques in lipofilling have been developed and these are now being tested to reconstruct and augment breasts. Over 500 surgical procedures have been carried out in France and Italy, where the fat cells are placed under the skin in tunnels but not in the breast tissue. The cells then grow and increase the volume of the breast. Although the changes still show up on mammograms, it has been found that experienced radiologists can differentiate these from cancer. Fat transfer does not result in a dramatic increase; in most cases it amounts to one cup size, but it does improve fullness in the upper part of the breast where it is most often lost with age.

Trials are now being conducted in the UK and a private clinic is offering the treatment.

COST: ABOUT £6,500.

A WORD OF WARNING
It's important to remember that cosmetic surgery is a time investment. Also, that it is an operation involving general anaesthetic and however brilliant your surgeon, there are always risks. Potential problems can include blood clots, infections or scarring not settling. You are almost certainly committing yourself to further surgery in the future as breast implants will probably need replacing. Manufacturers' life expectancy for implants is generally ten to fifteen years, although they may last longer.

MUMMY MAKEOVER

The mummy makeover corrects the changes that result from pregnancy and breastfeeding. The procedure rebuilds the breasts using breast augmentation as well as lifting and reshaping.

Damage to the tummy is corrected with a direct repair of the split in the abdominal rectus muscles as well as a removal of extra skin and fat in the lower half of the tummy.

RECOVERY AND COMPLICATIONS

This is major surgery and recovery would be the same as for a combined breast augmentation, uplift and tummy tuck. Complete rest would be advised for the first couple of weeks with a downtime of around six weeks, avoiding exercise, bending or lifting.

COST: FROM £13,500.

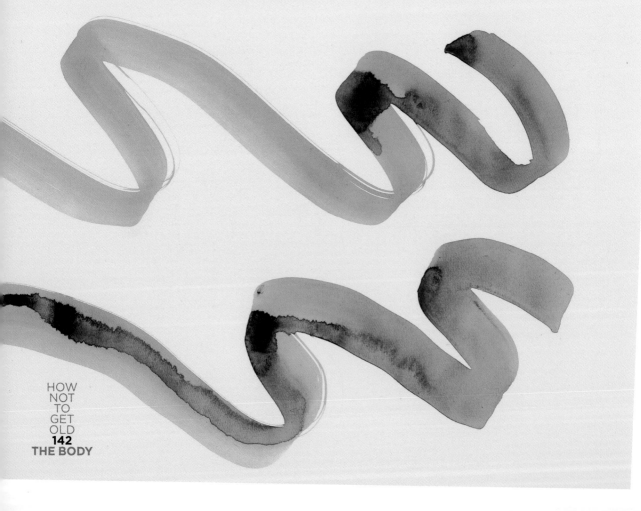

HOW
NOT
TO
GET
OLD
142
THE BODY

LAUREN'S STORY

Lauren is a care worker living in Kent. Over the course of a year she lost 6 stone through a combination of a healthy diet and exercise. She walked everywhere, took Zumba classes and has maintained a steady weight of 9 stone 2 pounds for over six months. She is sensible about what she eats and continues to exercise. She looks like the young twenty-five year old she is – until she gets undressed. The weight loss has left her with excess skin and sagging breasts that no amount of exercise will put right. 'My body looks more like the elderly people I work with,' she says.

Lauren would like the confidence to swim and go to the beach, to wear the clothes her friends wear. Basically she would like to feel good about herself and comfortable in her own skin. She is not interested in any other cosmetic procedures but feels that a breast uplift and implant together with a tummy tuck are her best options for dealing with the excess skin.

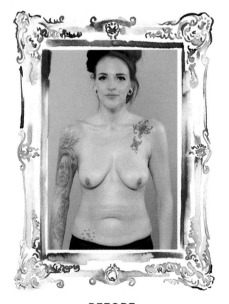

BEFORE

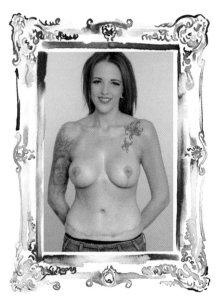

AFTER

HOW
NOT
TO
GET
OLD
143
THE BODY

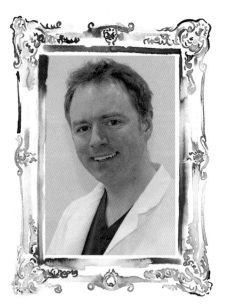

EXPERT PROFILE
MR STEPHEN HAMILTON

Mr Hamilton has been a consultant surgeon for eight years and worked in plastic surgery for around sixteen years. He realized when he was at medical school that he was interested in becoming a surgeon but it was watching a complex breast reconstruction that decided his field of expertise. 'There is no hiding behind plastic surgery, your work is there to be seen. It combines art and surgery in one.' Seeing the enormous difference that surgery can make to someone's life, both medically and psychologically, means that he has never regretted his choice of career.

Alongside his private cosmetic and reconstructive practice, Mr Hamilton also works as a consultant plastic surgeon and Clinical Director of Plastic Surgery, Breast Surgery and Dermatology at the Royal Free Hospital in London. He is a member of the GMC's Specialist Register in Plastic Surgery and a full member of the British Association of Plastic Reconstructive and Aesthetic Surgeons (BAPRAS) and the British Association of Aesthetic Plastic Surgeons (BAAPS).

Mr Hamilton's advice to anyone considering cosmetic surgery is to take plenty of time with your surgeon to discuss every detail. He has refused potential patients if he thinks they have made a spur-of-the-moment decision. He always shows pictures of his work, and tries to give sensible advice, making sure people have weighed up all the consequences, and that their expectations and motivations for going ahead are realistic.

A lot of his work is in post-cancer breast reconstruction, which often uses tummy tissue so there is a link between the two types of surgery he is performing on Lauren.

HOW
NOT
TO
GET
OLD
144
THE BODY

SURGERY

Stephen has decided to use 300-g round implants. The breast augmentation, mastopexy (lift) and abdominoplasty (tummy tuck) will all be carried out at the same time, taking around four hours altogether. Lauren will then spend two nights in hospital.

RECOVERY

Lauren will need to sleep upright for the first night and then propped up on an extra pillow for the next two weeks. She will wear support garments for six weeks and must not do any exercise or heavy lifting during that time. After the first two weeks most of the dressings and tapes will be removed and she should then keep reasonably active, although she should avoid anything strenuous. The tightness in the tummy lasts for around two weeks and can make it difficult to straighten up completely.

Moisturizing and massaging the scars with silicon gels and oils can help but Lauren will be given detailed information about this.

SCARRING

This can be fairly extensive for the tummy tuck – it is usually longer than a caesarean scar, for instance, and there will be an extra scar around the belly button. For the breasts there will be a periareolar scar with a vertical scar running down to the chest. In plastic surgery generally, surgeons always try to hide scars as far as possible.

HOW
NOT
TO
GET
OLD
145
THE BODY

WHAT WOULD I LOOK LIKE?

Ever wondered what you'd look like with bigger boobs, a different-shaped nose or a tighter tummy? Even if you're not seriously considering changing anything, most people occasionally look in the mirror and ask 'what if...'

On *How Not To Get Old* contributors have been offered the chance to see exactly how they would look through use of the Vectra 3D Imaging System. The digital scanner analyses their face or body to show exactly what they look like now and the difference that various surgical or non-surgical procedures could make to their appearance.

Nick Miedzianowski-Sinclair who operates the system at the Cosmetic Imaging Studio believes that it can really help people make informed decisions about what they want. And in practice he often finds that after seeing what they would look like, many of his clients choose not to go ahead with a procedure.

The 3D Imaging provides people with a 180-degree image of their face or breasts, and a 360-degree image of their body, which is then manipulated. For the face it can demonstrate the effect of various procedures including face and brow lifts, eyelid surgery, fillers and facial contouring. For anyone considering breast augmentation or a breast lift, it can show what different-sized implants would realistically look like on them, which is very different from seeing a certain cup size on someone else. In terms of the body, the 360-degree image helps to assess what could be achieved through a tummy tuck, liposuction, buttock shaping and cellulite treatment.

'It helps to take away some of the guesswork and allows people to define their treatment goals and assess exactly what could be achieved,' Nick explained. 'It gives people the confidence to know what they want and to be able to show this to their surgeon.'

Alongside 3D imaging, the clinic also offers skin analysis. This will assess sun and capillary damage, pigmentation and wrinkles to give a clear idea of skin condition and any underlying problems, so that treatment can be better targeted.

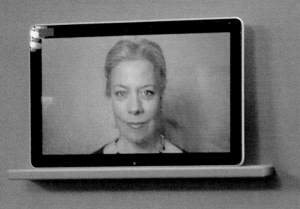
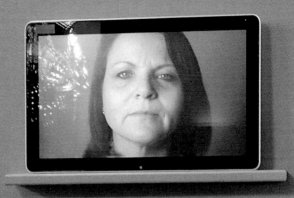
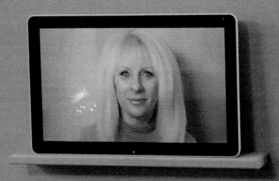
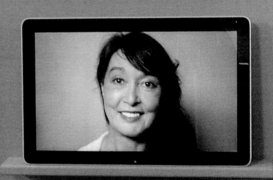
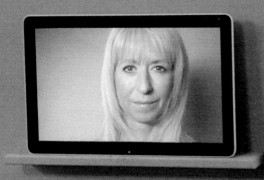
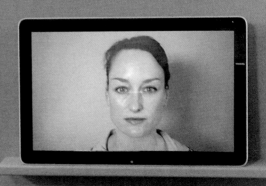

TUMMIES

Problems with excess skin on the abdomen are usually caused by pregnancy, where the muscles may also be weakened or even pulled apart, and by dramatic weight loss. Skin may also be affected by stretch marks which are the result of extreme stretching through pregnancy or weight fluctuations.

TUMMY TUCK (ABDOMINOPLASTY)

There are different procedures available:

◉ STANDARD TUMMY TUCK Excess fat and skin between the pubic area and navel are removed. Patients are left with a long, usually curved scar from hip to hip across the lower part of the abdomen, level with the pubic hair. There will also be a scar around the belly button. Any looseness or problems with the muscles of the abdominal wall are repaired at the same time. Liposuction is sometimes carried out in conjunction with the operation.

◉ MINI-TUCK Surplus skin below the belly button is removed, leaving a low scar across the pubic area but no scar around the navel. Liposuction is normally needed at the same time to reduce the layer of fat.

◉ EXTENDED TUCK The procedure is extended around to the back and lower sides, resulting in a very extensive scar.

◉ ENDOSCOPIC ABDOMINOPLASTY Keyhole surgery through a small incision just above the pubic hair is used to tighten the muscles of the abdomen. No skin is removed but liposuction may be carried out at the same time.

RECOVERY AND COMPLICATIONS
A standard tummy tuck is a serious operation requiring at least two days stay in hospital. Drains are inserted, dressings will be needed for at least two weeks, sometimes more, and the stomach can feel very tight at first, making it hard to straighten up. Patients are usually advised to wear support garments for six weeks and must avoid any bending, lifting or exercise during that time.

All the normal complications associated with major surgery apply here, including deep vein thrombosis and pulmonary embolism. Follow-up surgery is sometimes needed plus liposuction.

COST: £5,000+ FOR A STANDARD TUMMY TUCK.

LOUISE'S STORY

Louise is twenty-eight and the mother of two young children aged seven and two. Following the birth of her second child she dropped from a size eighteen to a size eight through a combination of healthy diet and exercise. She blames the combination of pregnancy and weight loss for her stomach, which she describes as, 'stretchy, loose, uneven and strange'. It doesn't matter how much she tries, nothing seems to help tone her tummy.

She is a confident young woman – having completed an economics and politics degree she is now a year into a law conversion course. She would now like to feel as confident about her body, to wear jeans and the sorts of clothes others her age can wear. Ultimately she would like not to feel self-conscious when she takes her children swimming or to the beach.

Louise has been advised that the only solution to deal with the loose, surplus skin on her stomach is a tummy tuck. She saw several different plastic surgeons and looked at examples of their work. She felt that Mr Richards stood out. He had a good reputation and was informative and professional. She particularly like the demonstration of care shown by him and his clinic.

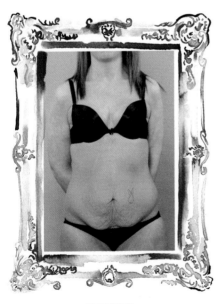

BEFORE

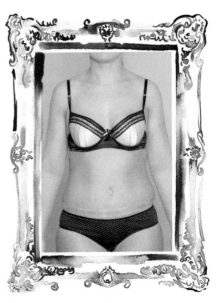

AFTER

HOW
NOT
TO
GET
OLD
149
THE BODY

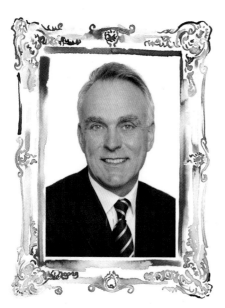

EXPERT PROFILE
MR ADRIAN RICHARDS

Mr Richards qualified as a doctor in 1988 and has specialized in plastic surgery for the past twelve years. He has extensive experience as a consultant plastic surgeon at Stoke Mandeville NHS Trust and is now surgical director at Aurora Clinics, a private practice.

Recognizing the demand for excellence from plastic surgeons, he frequently collaborates with other leading plastic surgeons worldwide to bring new surgical and non-surgical innovations to his practice. He sees meeting new patients and helping them achieve the results they want as one of the highlights of his job.

Mr Richards specializes in facial rejuvenation and breast surgery and has had considerable media attention. He is the founder of Cosmetic Courses, accredited by the Royal College of Physicians, which offers training to medical practitioners wanting to enter the aesthetics market. He was also the lead investigator in recent research into the use of Botox® for cosmetic purposes.

He is fully registered with the General Medical Council and is a member of the British Association of Plastic and Reconstructive Surgeons (BAPRAS), the British Association of Aesthetic Plastic Surgeons (BAAPS), and the International Society of Aesthetic Plastic Surgery (ISAPS).

HOW
NOT
TO
GET
OLD
150
THE BODY

TREATMENT

Louise has opted for a standard tummy tuck to remove excess skin and repair the muscles of her abdomen, which split during pregnancy. With two children to care for she has gone into every detail of her operation and recovery extremely carefully.

★ She has been told that she must rest completely for the first week and should expect to take between four and six weeks off work.

★ For the first week she must sleep sitting up and after that should be careful to sleep propped up with a pillow under her knees.

★ After any surgery or general anaesthetic, the head-above-heart rule applies to keep blood pressure steady.

★ She must be careful about bathing and cannot shower for the first week.

★ She must wear a support corset for four to six weeks and avoid lifting or exercise.

★ She won't be able to drive for ten days.

★ It's not unusual for patients to feel depressed or down during the recovery period.

In the longer term, Louise knows she has to be serious about aftercare. Surgery to the abdomen and muscles affect the back and posture; total repair is likely to take around a year. She has also been warned to avoid the sun for at least a year to allow the scar time to heal. In addition, should she decide to have more children, she knows she would almost certainly need a mini repair.

HOW
NOT
TO
GET
OLD
151
THE BODY

UPPER BODY LIFT

Upper body lifts are most often carried out after significant weight loss. The surgeon creates a belt-like incision at the bra line. He then performs a combination of procedures including a tummy tuck, liposuction, and removal of excess skin.

Drainage tubes are inserted and must be kept in place for two weeks. There is likely to be significant scarring.

RECOVERY AND COMPLICATIONS

This is a major surgical procedure involving a two-night stay in hospital. Complications include all the problems associated with abdominoplasty and major operations generally. You should expect at least eight weeks downtime.

COST: FROM £6,500.

LOWER BODY LIFT (BELT LIPECTOMY)

Like the upper body lift, this is most often performed after significant weight loss.

The lower half of the body is literally lifted as the surgeon creates a belt-like incision above the buttock and outer thighs. He then carries out a combination of procedures including a tummy tuck, liposuction and removal of excess skin.

Drainage tubes remain in place for two weeks and there is likely to be considerable scarring.

RECOVERY AND COMPLICATIONS

Recovery and risks are the same as for the upper body lift. Again, you should expect to remain in hospital for at least two days, with a minimum of eight weeks recovery time.

COST: FROM £6,500.

LIPOSUCTION

Liposuction, also known as liposculpture and suction-assisted lipectomy, is a fat removal technique that involves inserting a narrow tube through a small incision into the problem area. The fat cells are broken up with a saline solution and removed through the tube. A strong vacuum pump provides suction, although a syringe can sometimes be used for small areas.

The procedure helps remove stubborn pockets of fat and permanently changes your body shape. Often used on the stomach alongside tummy tucks, it can be used on virtually any area of the body that tends to accumulate fat, including arms, chin, neck, hips, back, knees, ankles, inner thighs, loins (or love handles) and chest.

BAAPS stresses that liposuction is not a treatment for general obesity; it can only be used on localized areas. Where skin has lost elasticity, it can also leave excess skin, which would need to be removed. Cellulite and wrinkles in the skin will also not be improved by the procedure.

RECOVERY
There can be extensive bruising which can be painful. This usually fades after a month but the lumpiness and swelling from deeper level bruising can last for up to six months. If legs have been treated, ankles can swell for a few weeks, and if the treatment is to the ankles they can remain swollen for some months. There is often some numbness in the treated area, which should disappear. There will also be small scars from the incisions. As a result of the swelling, the full effects of the treatment will not be seen for some months.

RESULTS
As fat cells are not thought to regenerate in adults, the results should be permanent.

COST: £1,500–£5,000.

HOW
NOT
TO
GET
OLD
153
THE BODY

NON-SURGICAL BODY TREATMENTS

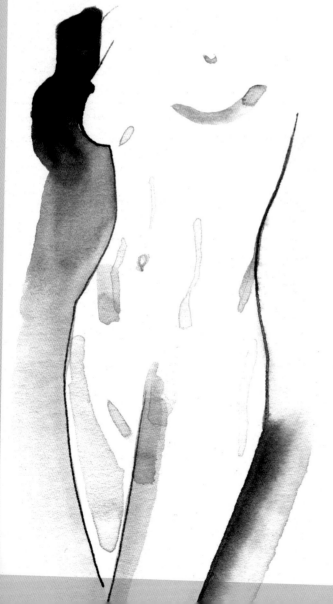

It is important not to overlook the body when it comes to anti-ageing treatments. And apart from the obvious exercise and diet, there's a lot that can be done. An increasing number of non-invasive rejuvenating treatments are now available to tackle those areas that don't respond easily to exercise and are a real giveaway when it comes to age.

COOLSCULPTING®

Dr Tracy Mountford, one of the UK's most sought-after cosmetic doctors, is particularly excited by developments in cryolipolysis. The name may sound futuristic, but she stresses there is strong science behind the treatment, which is more generally known as CoolSculpting.

Developed by Harvard scientists, CoolSculpting is a patented, clinically proven, FDA-approved body-contouring treatment. The procedure freezes fat cells to eliminate stubborn areas of fat without damage to the skin. It is suitable for men and women of all ages and typically patients see approximately 30 per cent reduction of fat in the treated area after one visit. Even more can be lost with additional sessions.

It is not a treatment for people who are generally overweight but it can be used to target specific areas such as muffin tops, love handles, post-pregnancy tummies, waists and stubborn menopausal bulges as well as back fat.

TREATMENT
The clinician positions the device on the body which then draws up the bulge to be treated between two cooling panels. The sensation is that of a firm pressure and enough of a pull to ensure the selected tissue will be cooled efficiently.

Patients are aware of intense cold but this soon fades and most patients spend the time reading or relaxing. During the treatment, fat cells are crystallized and then naturally eliminated from the body over a short period.

Each area takes one hour to treat and there's usually little, if any, recovery time, so patients can return to normal activities straight away.

RESULTS
Changes may be visible just three weeks after treatment, although patients will experience the most dramatic results between eight and twelve weeks later. However the body will still be flushing out fat cells and will continue to do so after the treatment.

The Cosmetic Skin Clinic where Dr Mountford practises has become the first clinic in Europe to offer Dual-Sculpting® which is patented to treat two areas at once by using two machines. The most impressive results can be seen with treatment to transformation, where a number of areas are treated in one session.

COST: VARIES ACCORDING
TO THE AREA TREATED
(AROUND £800 PER AREA).

HOW
NOT
TO
GET
OLD
155
THE BODY

THERMAGE® RADIOFREQUENCY SKIN TIGHTENING

Also recommended by Dr Mountford, Thermage is an FDA-approved, non-invasive procedure that has been clinically proven to help smooth, tighten and contour skin to give a rejuvenated, younger appearance. It delivers heat deep into the layers of skin to tighten existing collagen and stimulate the natural formation of new collagen over time, reducing sagging and improving the texture of the skin surface.

It has been used successfully for some years to treat the face, including jawline, eyes and forehead. The improved Comfort Pulse Technology not only makes it more comfortable, it is also suitable for tightening crepey, sagging skin on the tummy, arms, thighs and buttocks.

TREATMENT

A hand piece with a smooth, flat tip delivers the radiofrequency. Multiple passes are made over the treatment area and there is a sensation of heat as energy is pulsed. The device monitors the temperature of the skin and applies a cooling spray before, during and after the application of heat. Many patients liken it to a deep, slightly hot massage.

There may be minimal redness afterwards but this generally disappears within hours and patients can return to normal activities immediately.

RESULTS

There is a noticeable difference immediately but it takes around twelve to sixteen weeks for the full effects to develop as collagen is renewed. Usually one treatment gives good results; a top-up treatment will be needed every two years.

COST: VARIES WIDELY ACCORDING TO THE AREA TREATED (AROUND £2,000 FULL FACE, £1,750 EYES).

Dr Mountford suggests that particularly useful anti-ageing treatments for the body include Thermage to tone and tighten tummies, arms, thighs and buttocks, and Microsclerotherapy to remove unsightly thread veins.

MICROSCLEROTHERAPY

Thread veins are small spidery purple or red veins that can develop anywhere on the body but are particularly common on the legs, from the top of the thigh to the ankle. Thread veins are not painful and don't pose any major health problems but many people find them unsightly and embarrassing – however smooth and toned your legs may be they seem to be a real sign of age.

Microsclerotherapy is a safe technique for removing thread veins which has been used in Europe for over forty years. It removes abnormal veins by fibrosing them to break them down. Side effects are few with minimal bruising.

After treatment, support hosiery is worn to provide compression for a few days afterwards. It usually takes more than one session depending upon the severity of the thread veins.

COST: FROM £150–£250 PER SESSION.

VELASHAPE®

Described as a non-surgical alternative to liposuction, Velashape uses a combination of radiofrequency, infrared light technology, massage and vacuum to tone and sculpt. It is said to boost the breakdown of fat and help lymphatic drainage and tightening as well as reducing cellulite on tummies, knees, thighs and bottom. Four weekly treatments are recommended to achieve the best results.

COST: £200 PER TREATMENT.

HOW
NOT
TO
GET
OLD
157
THE BODY

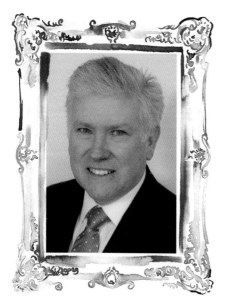

EXPERT PROFILE
MR CHRISTOPHER INGLEFIELD

After gaining his medical degree at the University of the West Indies in Jamaica and Trinidad, Mr Inglefield completed his specialist surgical training in the UK, going on to become a Plastic Reconstructive and Cosmetic Surgeon.

Mr Inglefield attends and speaks at conferences and workshops all over the world and has written and contributed to many specialist books. He is a member of the International Society of Aesthetic Plastic Surgery (ISAPS), the UK Association of Aesthetic Plastic Surgery (UKAAPS), the World Professional Association for TransGender Health, the Caribbean Association of Plastic and Reconstructive Surgeons, the British Burn Association, the British Microsurgical Society, the International Federation for Adipose Therapeutics and Science (IFATS), the British Association of Surgical Oncology and the Royal Society of Medicine – Plastic Surgery Section.

THE TREATMENT – RECELL

ReCell is one of the innovative treatments Mr Inglefield offers. It enables a surgeon to apply skin cells, collected from a small sample of the patient's own skin, to an area that needs new cells to ensure appropriate healing. It is used to treat skin defects, to accelerate healing, minimize scarring and reintroduce normal skin colour and pigment to skin. It can be used in a wide variety of wound, burn, plastic, reconstructive and cosmetic procedures, treating old scars, stretch marks and even for tattoo removal.

HOW IT WORKS

The patient's skin cells are harvested from a biopsy (often taken from behind the ear) and contain 'building block' cells to promote healing and cells that give skin its colour. A suspension is produced containing the skin cells, which is then sprayed on to scars, burns, wounds, areas of hyperpigmentation or excess whiteness where they multiply and create new healthy skin tissue. Because the new cells are grown from a patient's own cells, there is no risk of rejection or disease. The simple spray application means treatment takes just a few minutes.

HOW
NOT
TO
GET
OLD
158
THE BODY

HISTORY

The spray-on autologous skin culture treatment was developed by Professor Fiona Wood and scientist Marie Stoner in 1994 and was routinely used to treat burns victims at the Royal Perth Hospital in Western Australia. Its incredible results were seen when it was used to treat the Bali terrorist bombing victims in 2002.

THE PROCEDURE

A small biopsy of skin is collected, preferably from an area close to the skin to be treated. This ensures the treated area has the same texture and colour as the surrounding skin. The patient will have a local anaesthetic to numb any discomfort. The biopsy is usually between one and two square centimetres in size and will also be treated with the ReCell spray to help it heal properly.

While the surgeon is preparing the area to be treated, the skin will be placed into the ReCell device which will separate the cells, allowing the surgeon to spray them on to the area to regenerate.

RECOVERY

After the operation the treated area and biopsy site will be covered with a dressing. The area will initially be numb but may sting soon after the operation. This is normal and the patient may take medication to reduce any discomfort.

After about a week the dressing will be removed by the doctor or clinic nurse; timing will depend upon the reason why ReCell has been used. The skin will be red and there may be some scabs. The doctor will give advice concerning what creams should be used and what can be expected after the treatment.

If the treatment has been to reintroduce pigment (for instance in conditions such as vitiligo), re-pigmentation will occur slowly over several months as the cells grow, mature and start to produce pigment, or melanin. It is normal for pigmentation to take some time to reach its optimum state.

RESULTS

Long-term results following surgery with ReCell very much depend upon the reason for undergoing treatment, the severity of the condition or wound, and the natural ability of the body to recuperate afterwards.

BODY TREATS

Soothing body treatments can put a spring in your step and help you feel and look younger. A professional massage can ease muscles, boost circulation and generally lift your mood. Choose from moisturizing, rejuvenating treatments, to invigorating ice therapies to improve lymphatic drainage, hot stones for deep treatment or aromatherapy to restore your body's equilibrium.

BODY WRAPS

Marine clay wraps are used to treat and tone tummies and thighs and are often combined with body brushing to assist lymphatic drainage and help detoxify the body and skin.

You are wrapped in clay-soaked bandages to compress fat and purge impurities externally through the skin and internally through the lymph system. Fatty tissue and skin should appear tighter and more toned afterwards, while any bloating from fluid retention is eased, resulting in a more contoured appearance.

As well as physical improvements, body wraps may help ease tension and improve sleep, giving a boost to low energy levels.

COST: FROM £100.

HOW
NOT
TO
GET
OLD
160
THE BODY

REFLEXOLOGY

Reflexology is a traditional treatment which applies pressure to reflex points on the feet to increase the circulation of blood flow and energy.

Grainy crystal deposits settle at nerve endings in the feet which are linked to different areas of the body; reflexology works to disperse these, improving circulation and flushing out toxins. As well as the feet, reflex points on the hands or ears can be worked which can be very relaxing.

COST: FROM £50 A SESSION, ALTHOUGH VARIES ACCORDING TO THE PRACTITIONER.

ACUPUNCTURE

Acupuncture is a traditional Chinese treatment and is among the oldest forms of healing practice in the world. It involves inserting and manipulating fine, sterile needles into specific points on the body which are associated with the flow of energy.

Acupuncture can be used to treat a variety of conditions, alleviating pain or discomfort, whether physical or mental, by rebalancing the body and allowing natural healing processes to take place.

It is a holistic treatment looking at the whole person and is used to help with a range of problems including stress, insomnia, fatigue, muscular and skeletal conditions and premature ageing.

COST: FROM £55 A SESSION, ALTHOUGH VARIES ACCORDING TO THE PRACTITIONER AND TREATMENT.

'ENJOY YOUR BODY. USE IT EVERY WAY YOU CAN. DON'T BE AFRAID OF IT OR OF WHAT OTHER PEOPLE THINK OF IT. IT'S THE GREATEST INSTRUMENT YOU'LL EVER OWN.'

MARY SCHMICH, *WEAR SUNSCREEN: A PRIMER FOR REAL LIFE*

HOW
NOT
TO
GET
OLD
161
THE BODY

NIPS AND TUCKS FROM AROUND THE WORLD

It is always interesting to see what's happening in other parts of the world and *How Not To Get Old* took a look at some of the current trends in cosmetic surgery. Some of the procedures they uncovered are frankly weird and unlikely to catch on here any time soon; a few just might signal the future of anti-ageing.

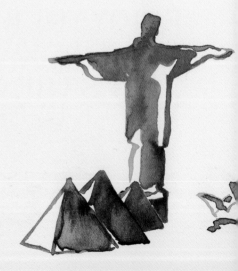

HOW
NOT
TO
GET
OLD
162
**NIPS AND
TUCKS FROM
AROUND
THE WORLD**

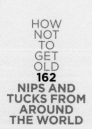

COSMETIC TREATMENTS

CHINA – MOXIBUSTION, TRADITIONAL CHINESE MEDICINE

This is a therapy using moxa, made from dried mugwort leaves. It plays an important role in the traditional medicines of China, Japan, Korea, Vietnam and Mongolia. Suppliers usually age the mugwort before grinding it to a soft fluffy mass. Practitioners burn the fluff or further process it into a cigar-shaped stick, to be applied to the patient's skin with the intention of stimulating circulation. It is said to encourage an overall feeling of youth.

CHINA – GUA SHA

An East Asian treatment technique in which a smooth, round-edged tool is stroked over the body to remove blood stagnation that can block the surface tissues, impeding organ and immune function. It offers various benefits including boosting the metabolism and flushing out cellular waste.

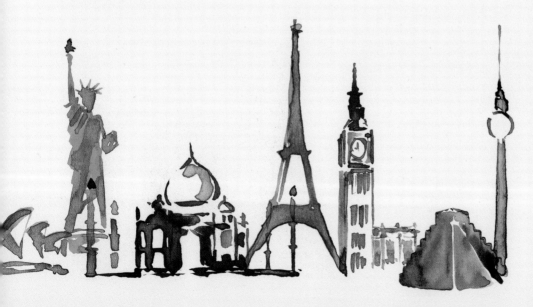

HOW
NOT
TO
GET
OLD
163
**NIPS AND
TUCKS FROM
AROUND
THE WORLD**

CZECH REPUBLIC – BEER BATHS

Taking the idea of a beer rinse for shiny hair a step further, a spa in the Czech Republic is offering visitors 'beer therapy' – a tub full of it. Visitors soak in the bath and reap the health benefits. It's supposedly anti-ageing and good for the skin.

HOLLAND – ANTI-WRINKLE TREATMENT

Developed by Dr Tom van Eijk, the Fern Pattern Technique is a specific method of injecting Restylane (a form of hyaluronic acid filler) from different angles and sides in the shape of a fern. This results in the Restylane being injected in the skin in multiple, tiny injections encouraging strength and elasticity and acting like a skin stiffening agent, rather than a simple filler which uses more material. The technique is used particularly to treat nasolabial smile lines between the nose and mouth.

JAPAN – JAPANESE BARBIE DOLL MAKE-UP

An internet craze where teenagers use make-up, including eye-enlarging contact lenses, to turn themselves into living versions of Licca-Chan, the Japanese equivalent of a Barbie doll.

JAPAN – 'YEABA' OR DOUBLE-TOOTH

Young women are paying hundreds of pounds for temporary or permanent caps designed to make their teeth look crooked, crowded and fang-like. The trend for 'yeaba', which can be translated as 'double-tooth' or 'snaggle-tooth', has proved surprisingly popular since it emerged in 2011. Japanese women are queuing up for the procedure, which they see as making them look younger, more attractive and more childlike.

RUSSIA – PLATZA, TRADITIONAL RUSSIAN MASSAGE

This alternative anti-ageing massage is designed to leave the client with youthful glowing skin, a strengthened metabolism, improved circulation and a relaxed mind. The traditional thermal massage is offered in Russian Turkish baths in a hot sauna-like room known as a 'schvitz' and involves the use of leafy, fragrant birch, oak or eucalyptus branches (or venik). A trained therapist shakes, brushes and presses the venik against the client's skin in sometimes vigorous circular movements, which may explain the glow. The treatment ends with a bucket of cold water being tipped over the client.

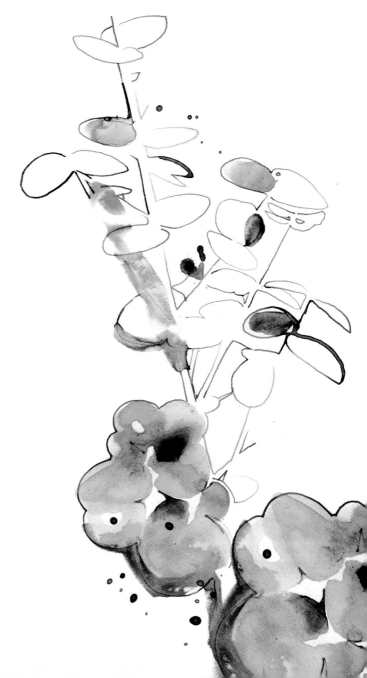

SURGICAL PROCEDURES

ARGENTINA – BLUGERMAN UMBILICOPLASTY TECHNIQUE

The problem of 'sad umbilicus' or excessive wrinkling around the belly button is fairly common after pregnancies or excessive fat aspiration during liposuction but it can be tricky to treat. Dr Blugerman has developed a technique for repair that involves no cutting of the stomach, just the use of needles, forceps and scissors.

ASIA – DOUBLE EYE LIFT

This is a popular procedure in Asia for those seeking a more Western look and also those who want to eradicate the drooping tired look that can come with age. According to BAAPS this is a very rare surgery in the UK.

BRAZIL – BUM LIFT

This is not unknown in the UK but in Brazil, along with liposuction and breast augmentation, it is more popular than facial procedures. Brazil is second only to the USA in terms of the number of cosmetic surgeries carried out each year. Brazil differs from the US and Europe, in that the emphasis is firmly on anti-ageing treatments for the body not the face.

TURKEY – BEARD AND CHEST HAIR RESTORATION

A full, rich beard and chest hair are viewed as signs of youth and success. This can be done in the UK but is rare according to BAAPS statistics.

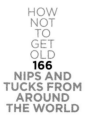
HOW
NOT
TO
GET
OLD
166
**NIPS AND
TUCKS FROM
AROUND
THE WORLD**

USA AND ASIA – LABIA MAJORA AUGMENTATION

This procedure involves plastic surgery to alter the inner and outer labia of women who are unhappy with the appearance of their genitals as they get older.

USA – HAIR RESTORATION ACELL/ENHANCED PRP HAIR RESCUE THERAPY

Developed by Dr Hitzig and Dr Prasad in New York, FDA-approved ACell wound healing powder is combined with the patient's platelet-rich plasma (PRP) to act as a hair growth accelerator and fertilizer. The ACell mesotherapy gun delivers the ACell product and PRP to the scalp, resulting in the growth of new hair, including terminal hairs in the original (non-grey) colour. This is definitely one to watch.

USA – WAIST RIB REMOVAL

This is an extremely complicated and controversial operation for those who are still dissatisfied with their waist size after a tummy tuck. It is one of the many procedures Valeria Lukyanova, the 'Human Barbie', is said to have undergone to make her body shape match the unrealistic dimensions of the doll. Some historians believe the Victorians were the first to remove ribs to allow for ever-tighter lacing of miniscule corsets in their desire for tiny waists. This is not a surgery that would be performed in the UK for cosmetic reasons and since the ribs protect some of the body's most vital organs it can be dangerous.

HOW
NOT
TO
GET
OLD
167
**NIPS AND
TUCKS FROM
AROUND
THE WORLD**

EXERCISE AND WELL-BEING

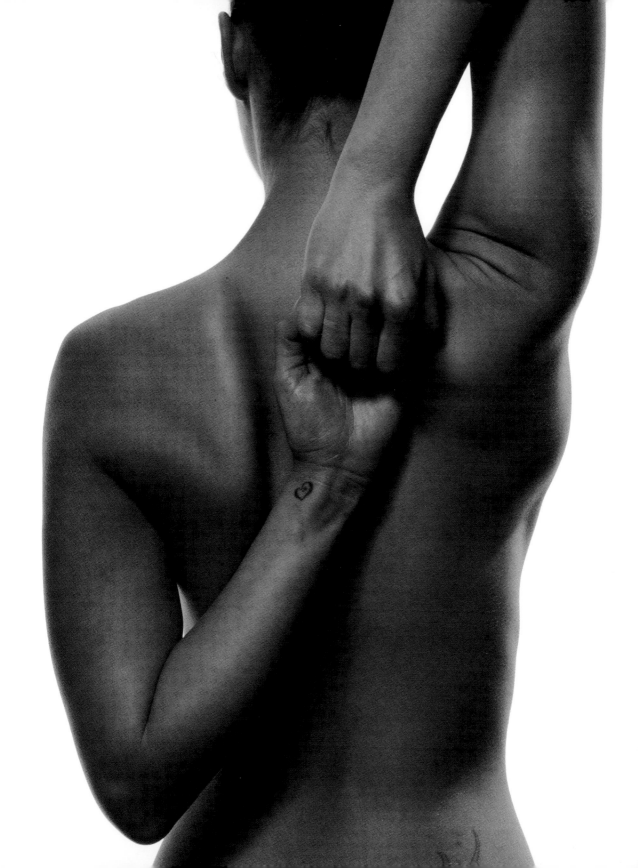

The outward signs that you're getting older are all too obvious. Everyone notices their own wrinkles, the skin that's beginning to sag on face and arms, the dimpled cellulite on thighs, the extra roll around the middle that's becoming ever more difficult to shift, but what's happening on the inside is just as dramatic.

It may be a cliché but the phrase 'use it or lose it' is all too true when it comes to the ageing body. There is, however, an easy way to halt the slide into old age, and that's simply to exercise. It doesn't have to be a strenuous workout or an energetic game of tennis – when it comes to exercise and well-being, there's something to suit everyone. You just have to keep moving to hold back the years.

MUSCLE MASS

Muscles make up about half your body weight and their condition and tone play a vital role in your level of strength and fitness, as well as your appearance. Lean muscle helps the body burn a greater number of calories but both muscle mass and metabolism decrease with the years and as we age our bodies need fewer calories to maintain the same weight.

BY THE TIME YOU ARE SEVENTY, YOUR MUSCLE STRENGTH WILL HAVE REDUCED BY A THIRD ON AVERAGE. REGULAR EXERCISE CAN PREVENT MUSCLE WASTAGE AND KEEP YOU TONED.

◎ MUSCLE MASS begins to decline from the early thirties onwards. On average women lose between 150–175 g (that's 5–6 ounces) of muscle mass each year and can gain the same or more in fat as their metabolism slows by up to 4 per cent a year.

◎ ALTHOUGH SOMEONE MAY WEIGH the same at sixty as they did at thirty, they are likely to have lost muscle. The muscle loss is not obvious because it will simply have been replaced by fat.

◎ MUSCLE LOSS dramatically increases after the menopause, perhaps linked to the loss of oestrogen.

◎ EXERCISE will help you to maintain as much muscle mass as possible.

◎ WITHOUT REGULAR EXERCISE, muscles simply waste away and can attract fluid, fat and toxins.

◎ THE HUMAN NUTRITION RESEARCH CENTER on Ageing at Tufts University, Boston, identified this process as *sarcopenia,* which translates as 'vanishing flesh'.

◎ WEIGHT-BEARING EXERCISES such as brisk walking, yoga, resistance training or lifting weights are among the most effective ways to build up lean muscle mass.

◎ TUFTS UNIVERSITY RESEARCH found that taking Vitamin E reduced free radical damage to muscles after exercise.

◎ PROTEIN AND AMINO ACIDS found in fish, meat and poultry all help to maintain muscle strength and suppleness.

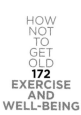
HOW
NOT
TO
GET
OLD
172
**EXERCISE
AND
WELL-BEING**

BONE DENSITY

Along with muscle mass, bone density can also decrease with age and from the mid-thirties the strength of bones and the connective tissue begins to deteriorate. In childhood the skeleton takes two years to completely renew itself; for an adult, the same process takes between seven and ten years.

◎ LACK OF OESTROGEN for women and testosterone for men accelerates the decline in bone density.

◎ BONE THINNING or osteoporosis is estimated to affect one in three women over the age of fifty. Over 230,000 fractures each year are linked to the condition.

◎ MAINTAINING A HEALTHY WEIGHT helps to ensure you get all the vital nutrients your skeleton needs and also avoids putting too much stress on joints and connective tissue.

◎ FISH OILS and glucosamine may help maintain cartilage and bones, neutralizing the effect of damaging enzymes.

HOW
NOT
TO
GET
OLD
173
**EXERCISE
AND
WELL-BEING**

◎ CALCIUM is vital for the formation and maintenance of healthy bones – good food sources are oily fish, dairy products, almonds and watercress. Calcium is particularly important for women. Research has shown that if there is insufficient calcium in the diet, women's bodies will simply take it from the bones, increasing the risk of osteoporosis.

◎ VITAMIN D is essential as calcium can only be properly absorbed alongside it. Your body can make its own Vitamin D from exposure to sunlight but a good food source is oily fish.

◎ EXERCISE has been shown to raise levels of testosterone and oestrogen which help calcium absorption. Regular exercise, particularly if it's weight-bearing, improves skeletal strength and helps to maintain healthy bone density.

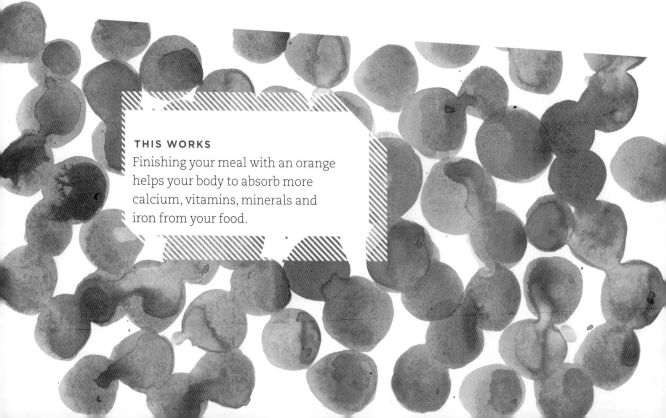

THIS WORKS
Finishing your meal with an orange helps your body to absorb more calcium, vitamins, minerals and iron from your food.

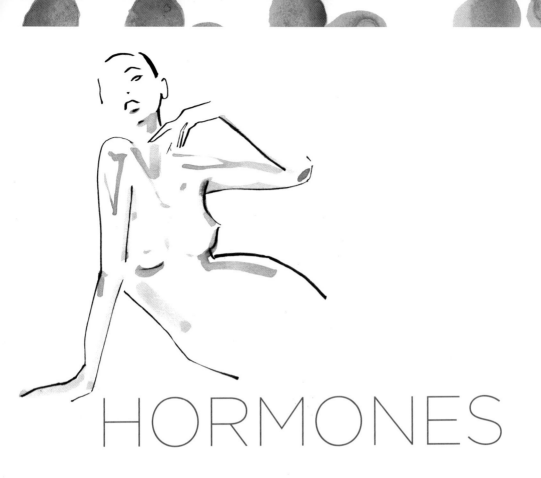

HORMONES

You can roll back years in terms of your body's muscle mass, bone density, strength and flexibility after just one year of regular resistance training. You should also find you have the metabolism, blood pressure and hormone levels of someone fifteen years younger.

Alongside muscle mass and bone density, the body's production of hormones also slows as we age. The drop in hormone levels is responsible for many of the obvious signs of ageing, from dry skin that wrinkles more easily, to dull hair, brittle nails and a further weakening of bones and loss of muscle strength.

HOW
NOT
TO
GET
OLD
175
**EXERCISE
AND
WELL-BEING**

◎ EXERCISE RELEASES ENDORPHINS, those feel-good hormones that lift your mood also reduce anxiety and hunger pangs. Just thirty minutes of exercise increases levels by 500 per cent and the effects will last up to eight hours.

◎ EXERCISE HELPS to raise natural levels of human growth hormone (or HGH) making you feel, look and think better. HGH plays a vital role in the repair of the skeleton and muscles, it helps to burn fat, boosts concentration levels and mood, improves sleep and helps skin hydration and texture. In other words increased HGH leaves you looking and feeling younger.

◎ LEVELS OF OESTROGEN are increased for up to four hours after exercise, improving your mood, metabolism and libido.

◎ TESTOSTERONE LEVELS rise for up to three hours following moderate exercise, improving self-confidence and sexual enjoyment as well as muscle tone and strength. As an added bonus, it reduces your body fat.

◎ THE PRODUCTION of other important hormones also increases after a workout, including glucagon which encourages the breakdown of fats, and insulin which regulates blood sugar levels.

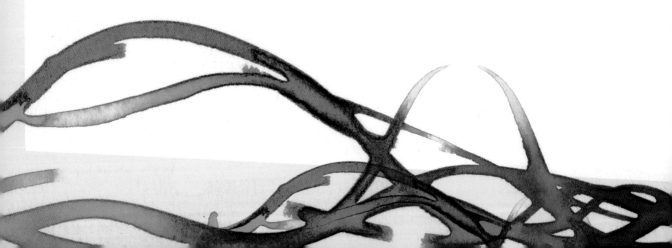

THE AGEING HORMONE

Unfortunately, the one hormone that increases with age is cortisol. A certain amount is essential: it's linked to adrenaline and the in-built 'fight or flight' response that takes over to get you out of danger. It also helps you to overcome any stressful situation. The problem is that large amounts can be harmful over time and the more stressed you are, the more cortisol your body produces, which in turn makes you even more anxious.

Cortisol is linked to the ageing process. High levels deplete the immune system, thin the skin and encourage wrinkles. It can also be the reason you feel tired all the time and even lead to you piling on weight. So, what can you do to bring cortisol levels down? Nothing is quite as effective as a good workout.

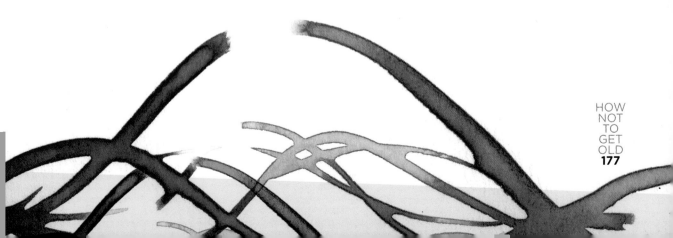

WAYS TO EXERCISE

It's important to think outside the box. If your heart sinks at the thought of high-tech Lycra sportswear and expensive gym membership then don't go there. Exercise should be fun and if it's going to be a regular feature of your daily life then it really has to be something you enjoy and not something you have to force yourself to do.

It helps to think about what you want to achieve. To look younger and feel fitter, plan activities to tackle different areas of your body. Aim to increase body strength, stamina and suppleness.

Walking, running, dancing and cycling will all raise your heart rate and make you breathe faster, improving aerobic fitness and stamina. Resistance training using a machine or the weight of your own body can all help body strength, while a Pilates or yoga workout will stretch and exercise your body to leave you supple and toned.

HOW
NOT
TO
GET
OLD
178
**EXERCISE
AND
WELL-BEING**

WHY RUN WHEN YOU CAN WALK?

Researchers at Lawrence Berkeley National Laboratory in California compared the general health of 33,060 runners and 15,945 walkers aged from eighteen to eighty. 'The more the runners ran, and the walkers walked, the better off they were in health benefits,' said Dr Paul Williams, the study leader. 'Run or walk and invest in your future health.'

More surprisingly, the researchers found that brisk walking brought all the health benefits of running and more without the risk of putting extra stress on the heart and joints. It's long been known that jogging and other high-impact exercise as you get older can exacerbate facial sagging and joint strain.

As long as people walked for long enough to use up the same amount of energy as they would running, their risk of heart disease, high blood pressure, diabetes and cholesterol all lowered. In fact, it was found that walking was more effective than running: walkers just had to do it for slightly longer. For instance, walking 4.3 miles would use as much energy as running for 3 miles but it would take around 38 minutes, rather than 15 minutes running.

WALKING THE DOG

Need a reason to go walking? Just get a dog. A recent survey found that the average British dog owner walks more than 500 miles a year exercising their pet. This amounts to an astounding 7,415 miles over a typical dog's lifetime – that's more than the distance from London to New York and back again.

And the health benefits don't stop there. Dog and cat owners live longer, suffer less stress and anxiety, have a reduced risk of depression, lower blood pressure and enjoy generally better emotional and physical health. The US Department of Health found that following a serious heart attack, 28 per cent of pet owners survived, compared with only 6 per cent who didn't own a pet. In addition, a 2008 study showed that cardiac patients who were pet owners recovered faster.

DID YOU KNOW?
VIBRATIONS FROM A CAT'S PURR CAN HELP RELIEVE PAIN.

YOGA

Yoga is really effective for lowering high cortisol levels. Aerobic-type exercise like running can put even more strain on the body if it is already stressed, while yoga achieves the opposite, helping to calm and focus your mind as well as toning and realigning muscles. There are many different styles of yoga, from the slower-paced Hatha, which takes you through a series of poses, to more vigorous styles such as Vinyasa or Ashtanga; the important thing is to find a class or instructor that suits you and your needs.

PILATES

Like yoga, Pilates aims to improve core strength and posture, while encouraging flexibility and tone. Dynamic Pilates is a more intense version aimed at slimming and building muscle tone by combining standard Pilates movements with weight and circuit training.

SHORT AND SWEET WORKOUTS

Short and sweet might not be quite the right description but fast and intense, certainly. It seems that four minutes of high-intensity circuit training can be more effective than a longer workout.

Dr Izumi Tabata, who worked as an adviser to Japan's Olympic speed skaters, found that an intense four-minute period of exercise followed by a ten-second rest period, repeated eight times, increases overall fitness, revives sluggish metabolisms and boosts circulation. The body burns fat faster and continues to do so for up to thirty-six hours after the workout. It also helps to stop your body craving sugary food.

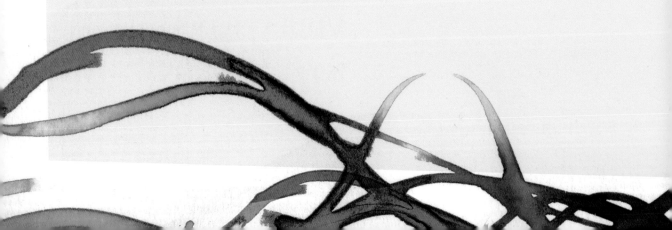

PERSONAL TRAINERS

Having your own personal trainer may seem like an expensive luxury but what about sharing a trainer with other people? Exercises can still be targeted to personal needs and there should be enough individual attention to make sure you're getting the most out of the time. Training with other people can encourage you to train harder and makes the whole experience more fun. There are a growing number of small group personal trainers who are making this an affordable option.

BOX FIT

Boxing – using a punch bag rather than an opponent – can be a wonderful way to release frustrations and get oxygen pumping through the system and to the brain, helping you feel less tired. Combined with circuit training at the gym, this can improve cardiovascular health and muscle strength.

BOOT CAMPS

If you're really after an intense short sharp shock to get you back on the fitness track, there are various types of 'boot camp' on offer. British Military Fitness run outdoor sessions across the UK, while many spas offer short residential boot camps where guests try a variety of activities with some one-to-one advice and instruction.

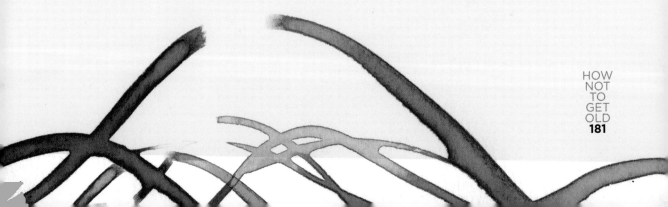

ALTERNATIVE WORKOUTS

There are some other activities you could try that provide a fantastic workout – and they don't even feel like exercise.

DANCE MAGIC

Zumba, with its infectious music, can give you a full body workout that doesn't feel like exercise; it lifts your mood and is a great stress buster. Experts reckon it usually takes three classes to become familiar with the repetitions in the dances and by then you'll be hooked. It engages muscles and tightens and tones your body, incorporating traditional fitness moves like lunges and squats, but in such a way that you don't notice you're doing them. It can be adapted to any fitness level and researchers calculate an hour of Zumba will burn an average of 800 calories.

And if Zumba isn't your thing, what about tap dancing, salsa, or whatever else appeals?

HOW
NOT
TO
GET
OLD
182
**EXERCISE
AND
WELL-BEING**

SKIP FOR JOY

Along with the hula hoop, dig out your old skipping rope for another fun activity from childhood that gives you a wonderful workout, too.

Skipping is cheap, effective, fat-burning and you can do it anywhere at a pace that suits you. Just ten minutes of skipping burns over 200 calories and has the same health benefits as a forty-five minute run, although skipping is far kinder to your joints. It provides a full body workout using core abdominal muscles, arm and legs, as well as improving flexibility, coordination and balance.

In terms of health, it lowers blood pressure and gives a boost to your circulation and cardiovascular system. Skipping is also a weight-bearing exercise so it is particularly good for the ageing body, improving muscle mass and bone density.

JOIN THE CHOIR

Singing is an aerobic activity that increases oxygen levels in the blood and exercises major muscle groups in your upper body – even when you're sitting down. Those are the findings of several studies, including one by Professor Graham Welch at the University of London who has looked at the developmental and medical aspects of singing over a period of thirty years.

It seems that singing lowers blood pressure and increases lung capacity, allowing you to breathe more easily. It also increases the sense of emotional well-being, reducing stress, encouraging serenity and may even help to rewire the brain after a stroke.

Singing alone in the shower or wherever the fancy takes you is good; singing with others is even better for your psychological health – production of the hormone oxytocin, the one that helps mothers and babies bond, soars when you sing with friends.

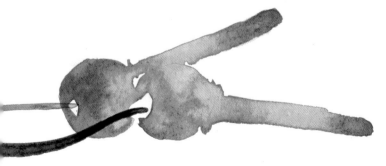

HOW
NOT
TO
GET
OLD
183
**EXERCISE
AND
WELL-BEING**

WAIST WHITTLER

Hula hoops were invented in 1958, sparking a craze that resurfaces every so often, for instance when Michelle Obama was photographed enthusiastically hula hooping with her daughters. And hooping is good for you.

The repetitive hip gyrations, swaying back and forward rather than in a circular motion, strengthen core muscles including the pelvic floor, abdomen and lower back, while at the same time tightening and toning your waist and bottom. It's estimated that hooping works around thirty muscles in and around your core, and may burn up to a hundred calories in just ten minutes. The list of benefits doesn't end there. It gives you an aerobic work out, improves your posture and, it's claimed, your sex life. Plus it's fun, makes you laugh (always a bonus) and leaves you feeling young again.

When it comes to hula hoops size matters. Basically the bigger you are the bigger the hoop should be. Standing with the hoop in front of you, the rim should come just above your navel. Hooper Street (www.hooperstreet.co.uk), which make hoops and offer classes and workshops, recommend a 1-metre (40-inch) hoop for most adults. Smaller hoops also make hooping harder, especially for beginners, while larger ones rotate more slowly.

Like any form of exercise, it's not advisable to start something new when pregnant or if you have a specific medical problem. Always consult your doctor first.

THIS WORKS
Exercising in the late afternoon or early evening will help you feel tired and sleep better at night.

HOW
NOT
TO
GET
OLD
184
**EXERCISE
AND
WELL-BEING**

LAUGH YOURSELF YOUNGER

A study of 54,000 Norwegians over a period of seven years found that those who had the most humorous outlook on life and laughed the most were likely to live longer. Taking the idea of laughter being the best medicine even further, Dr Madan Kataria has devised a system of Laughter Yoga to teach you to laugh for no reason. It apparently expands lung capacity and clears sinuses.

TALKING ITALIAN

It's not just your body that benefits from exercise. It has long been claimed that regularly tackling Sudoku and crossword puzzles helps guard against dementia but did you know that learning and speaking a foreign language can have the same effect? Doctors from York University in Toronto found that practising another language improved cognitive control, boosted brainpower and significantly slowed the onset of dementia.

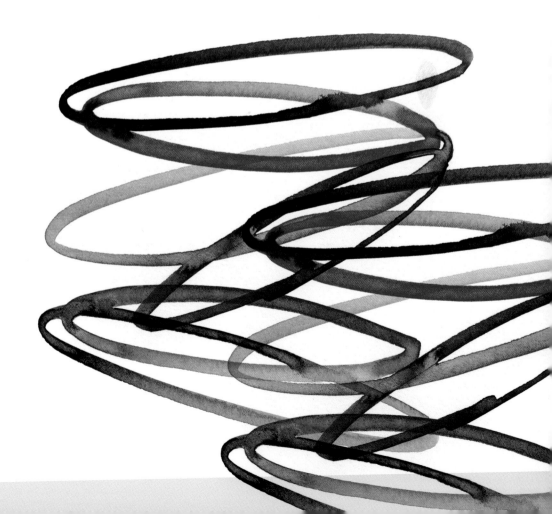

SWEET DREAMS

A healthy body needs a healthy mind and it's important to find time to clear your head of clutter, relax and feel good. Unwinding at the end of a busy day will also help you to sleep better.

A good night's sleep is vital for helping you to look younger and feel energized. While you sleep, your body repairs and restores itself, counteracting the ageing effects of stress and cortisol, and increasing its production of anti-ageing growth hormones.

However, the older we get, the longer it tends to take us to fall asleep and the less sleep we actually need. Far from being a cause for concern, it seems that you can have too much of a good thing. Research at the Scripps Sleep Center in California found that people who sleep between six and a half and seven and a half hours a night live the longest.

HOW
NOT
TO
GET
OLD
186
**EXERCISE
AND
WELL-BEING**

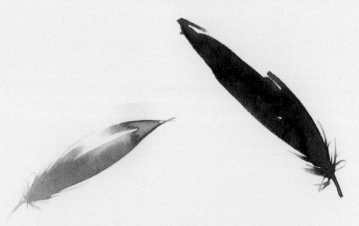

While sleeping too long may be bad, a lack of sleep has been linked to all sorts of health problems, weight gain and an increased risk of diabetes and heart problems. Insufficient sleep is also thought to lead to psychological conditions including depression and substance abuse, not to mention problems of concentration and memory.

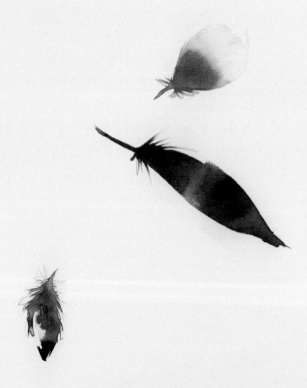

HOW
NOT
TO
GET
OLD
187
**EXERCISE
AND
WELL-BEING**

THE RHYTHM OF SLEEP

So how do you make sure you get the right amount to function at your best and wake feeling alert and ready to face the day ahead?

Researchers suggest there are two main factors to consider: basal sleep which is the amount of sleep our bodies require regularly to perform properly, and sleep debt, which is the sleep lost due to disturbed nights and poor sleep habits. Unfortunately, sleep debt builds up so although you may have had the right amount of basic basal sleep for several nights in a row you may still not have made up your sleep debt, which can be the reason why you still feel tired.

Add into this the issue of circadian dips – the points in any twenty-four hour period when you are programmed to feel sleepy and less alert, typically during the night and mid-afternoon – and it's no wonder you find yourself nodding off after lunch or when you sit down.

ONE IN THREE PEOPLE
WILL SUFFER FROM INSOMNIA
AT SOME POINT IN THEIR LIVES.

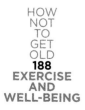
HOW
NOT
TO
GET
OLD
188
**EXERCISE
AND
WELL-BEING**

The good news is that sleep researchers believe that sleep debt can be 'paid off' – you just need to get into a healthy sleep pattern, scheduling sleep time as you would any other activity. The National Sleep Foundation has a wealth of information and recommendations on how to get a good night's rest.

◎ KEEP REGULAR HOURS for bedtime and waking, even at weekends.

◎ A RELAXING BEDTIME ROUTINE such as a warm bath with a few drops of lavender or chamomile oil added and relaxing music can really help.

◎ MAKE SURE your bedroom is quiet, dark and uncluttered.

◎ YOU WILL SLEEP BETTER if the room is cool rather than too hot.

◎ A SUPPORTIVE, comfortable mattress and pillows make a big difference.

◎ USE YOUR BEDROOM only for sleep (and sex).

◎ STUDIES HAVE FOUND that watching TV and using mobile phones and laptops inhibits relaxation and leads to disturbed sleep.

◎ AVOID EATING TOO LATE. Try to allow at least two to three hours before you go to bed.

◎ DON'T GO TO BED HUNGRY as low blood sugar levels will stop your body from producing sleep-promoting hormones.

◎ ALCOHOL may seem to help you sleep, but it's likely to wake you in the middle of the night when it prompts a burst of norepinephrine, a hormone that can jolt you awake and keep you restlessly tossing and turning for hours.

HOW
NOT
TO
GET
OLD
189
**EXERCISE
AND
WELL-BEING**

ANTI-AGEING FOOD

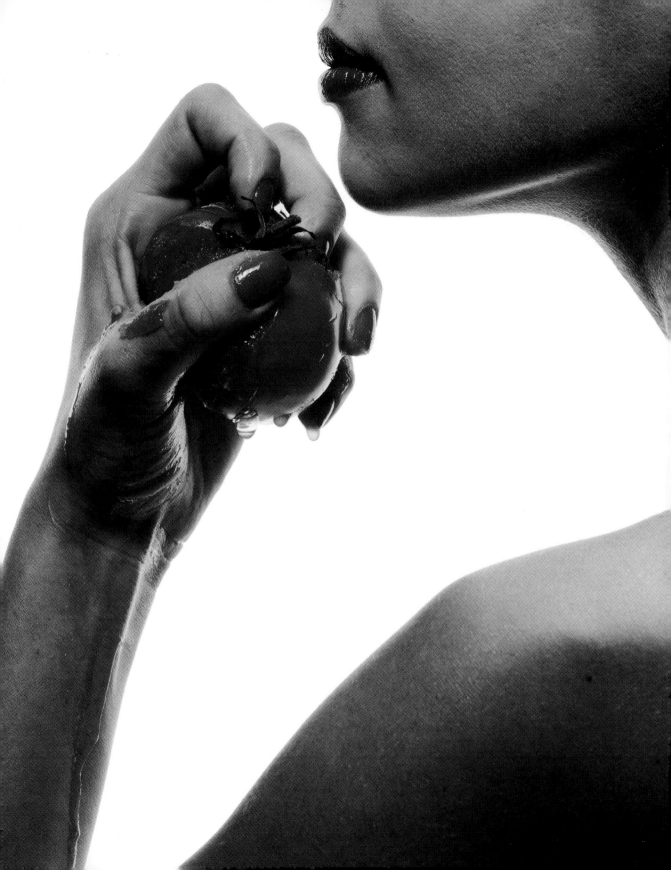

You're careful about skincare, you always wear sun protection, you're looking after your body, exercising and keeping active – you may even get the recommended seven hours' sleep each night – but if you really want to know how not to get old, you also need to know how to eat well to stay young. Choosing the right foods will supply your body with the right fuel it needs to really help slow the signs of ageing, building your health from the inside out.

KNOW YOUR NUTRIENTS

To an extent superfoods come and go. That's a gross overstatement, but there are definitely trends when it comes to healthy eating. One year everyone is raving about pomegranates and the berry of choice is blue, the next beetroot is the answer to boosting your heart health and detoxifying your system; recently 'cauliflower steak' has become the go-to vegetable. Then there are all the oils, grains and juices said to do wonders for your health. It can be hard to know what to believe.

The answer is that these are all still superfoods but it's the nutrients they contain that are key when it comes to choosing food to help keep you looking young.

A balanced, anti-ageing diet should include a combination of all of these vital nutrients:

◎ Essential fatty acids
◎ Antioxidants (including vitamins)
◎ Minerals
◎ Proteins

HOW
NOT
TO
GET
OLD
193
**ANTI-AGEING
FOOD**

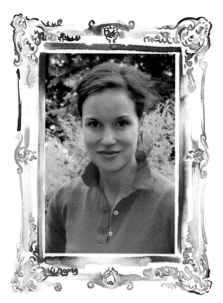

EXPERT PROFILE
ELIZABETH PEYTON-JONES

In the television series, Elizabeth Peyton-Jones, healthy eating and Youthing Guru, met Louise Redknapp to look at anti-ageing foods. For Elizabeth 'youthing' is something that is totally within your control. If you look in the mirror and see yellow eyes, wrinkles, dry or red skin it is usually as a direct result of what you are putting into your body. She firmly believes that you can make a visible difference and feel younger and more energetic by changing the way you eat.

If she had to point the finger at one main culprit when it comes to ageing she would blame inflammation. By this, she does not just mean the sort of inflammation you can see but the sort that affects skin, joints, the brain and your whole body. Inflammation is basically the body's reaction to any kind of allergen and it can show itself in auto-immune responses, sinusitis, candida, thinning hair and nails, dull eyes as well as muscle and bone loss.

'If the body is inflamed, the ageing process is accelerated.' Any anti-ageing diet should be targeted at reducing inflammation throughout the body, restoring balance.

In her excellent book *Eat Yourself Young*, she outlines her simple steps to a younger, healthier you:

HOW
NOT
TO
GET
OLD
194
ANTI-AGEING
FOOD

★ Eating fruit and vegetables that are 60–70 per cent water to keep you hydrated and alkalized. Cucumbers for instance are fantastic and lemons – perhaps surprisingly – are probably the best for counteracting acidity.

★ Foods that are high in Omega-3 and spices such as turmeric and ginger are excellent anti-inflammatories.

★ Important antioxidants will automatically be part of your daily diet if you are eating a wide variety of vegetables. Red beans, including kidney, aduki and pinto are particularly helpful.

★ Hormone-balancing foods are also important and can help reduce inflammation, which affects hormone production. Elizabeth is a huge fan of garlic – great for 'youthing' skin, it is also an antioxidant and helps to lessen the symptoms of falling levels of testosterone and oestrogen as we age.

Elizabeth advises limiting the following:

★ Packaged foods
★ Bad fats
★ Refined sugars
★ Too much salt

If you are really getting the anti-inflammatory nutrients you need, you will look brighter and younger but you will also feel energized. You will be calm and your memory will improve.

Elizabeth speaks from experience. She is a herbalist and naturopath who has run a natural healing practice in West London for the last fifteen years. She has seen for herself how a simple detox can make people seem physically and mentally younger. Once the allergens causing inflammation are removed, everything about a person changes, from attitude to looks. Her clients, who include models, actors and celebrities, have changed their lives in just a couple of months.

'People worry about the signs of ageing that are due to disease. It's the disease you need to stop not the age.'

ESSENTIAL FATTY ACIDS

Fat is good for you, or more precisely, the right kind of fat is good for you. Essential fatty acids, or EFAs, are fats that are essential for health but are not actually manufactured by our bodies, which means we have to include them in our diet. Good food sources include nuts, seeds, fish and seed oils and oily fish. They offer vital anti-inflammatory protection, reduce cholesterol levels, and stimulate and support the immune system.

Looks-wise, a lack of essential fatty acids results in dry, dehydrated, ageing skin and a tendency to put on weight. You need EFAs to kick-start your metabolism, to help you burn calories and to keep you feeling satisfied for longer.

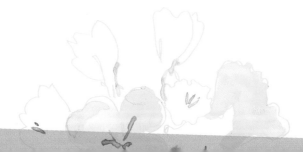

HOW
NOT
TO
GET
OLD
196
**ANTI-AGEING
FOOD**

OMEGA-6

In a balanced diet, linoleic acid is synthesized with EPA from Omega-3 to form prostaglandins, vital for normal body functions, as well as preventing blood clots, lowering blood pressure, reducing inflammation and boosting the immune system.

GOOD FOOD SOURCES FOR OMEGA-6 INCLUDE

Blackcurrant seed oil
Borage oil
Chicken
Evening primrose oil
Flax seeds and oil
Hemp seeds
Olives and olive oil
Pine nuts
Pistachios
Pumpkin seeds

IT'S ALL IN THE BALANCE
A healthy diet needs the right balance between Omega-3 and Omega-6. Nutritionists usually recommend twice as much Omega-6 as Omega-3.

The problem is that many Western diets rely too heavily on meat and dairy products, leading to an overload of Omega-6 which can then suppress the absorption of Omega-3. This creates a vicious circle, as without sufficient Omega-3 the body cannot utilize the beneficial properties of Omega-6. Researchers believe this is one of the main reasons for the growing rates of inflammatory disorders.

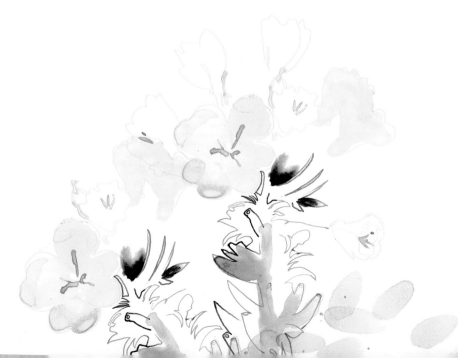

OMEGA-3

The three major types important
for health are:

ALA (alpha-linolenic acid)
DHA (docosahexaenoic acid)
EPA (eicosapentaenoic acid)

Research has shown that Omega-3 fatty
acids can help prevent heart disease,
strokes, diabetes and arthritis, as well
as reduce inflammation, improve brain
function and control insulin levels and
excess weight. A lack of them has been
associated with problems of depression.
They are also thought to be helpful in
targeting the compounds which cause
allergic reactions and skin conditions.
Most recently, studies have suggested
that EPA is the really important one
to look out for.

FOODS RICH IN OMEGA-3 INCLUDE
Anchovies
Avocados
Crab
Fish oils
Flax seeds and oil
Hemp seeds and oil
Herring
Mackerel
Pilchards (including tinned)
Pumpkin seeds
Salmon
Sardines (including tinned)
Soya products
Trout
Tuna (fresh, not tinned)
Walnuts and oil
Whitebait

Always look for unrefined, unprocessed
oils as Omega-3 can be damaged through
processing and cooking. The Omega-3
found in vegetable sources has to be
converted to DHA and EPA by the body,
whereas most of the Omega-3 in fish
and fish oils is already in that form.

HOW
NOT
TO
GET
OLD
198
**ANTI-AGEING
FOOD**

OILY FISH

As well as providing a hefty dose of Omega-3, fish also contain the chemical compound DMAE (dimethylaminoethanol), which is said to help concentration and mood, boosting mental alertness. It is also suggested that it can counteract the signs of ageing in skin, improving tone and firmness. The best food sources are wild salmon and sardines.

EXPERT ADVICE

The best way to ensure you are getting all the Omega-3 you need is through diet. The National Institute for Clinical Excellence (NICE) recommends eating at least two portions of oily cold-water fish, such as salmon and sardines, each week.

Due to the pollutants that can be found in some varieties of oily fish, pregnant women and those who are breastfeeding are recommended to eat no more than two portions a week.

DID YOU KNOW?

IF YOU DON'T EAT FISH, HEMP OIL IS A GOOD SOURCE OF OMEGA-3. IT CONTAINS MORE ESSENTIAL FATTY ACIDS THAN FLAX SEED OIL AND IS RICH IN ANTIOXIDANT VITAMIN E, WHICH IS GOOD FOR YOUNG-LOOKING SKIN.

OMEGA-9

This is not strictly an essential fatty acid as the body can make a small amount itself. It is a monounsaturated fatty acid also known as oleic acid.

Omega-9 helps fight inflammation, maintains blood sugar balance, boosts the immune system and helps prevent the build-up of fatty deposits in the arteries. It also helps to maintain a youthful complexion.

FOODS RICH IN OMEGA-9 INCLUDE
Avocados
Berries
Olives and olive oil
Peanuts
Pecans

EXPERT ADVICE

When looking for a supplement to boost your intake of essential fatty acids, look at the list of ingredients and make sure it contains EPA Omega-3. Recent research suggests 1000 mg a day is the optimum dose. Cheaper supplements may not deliver and can work out to be more expensive in reality when you work out how much you'd have to take. Most people will not need to supplement their Omegas 6 or 9.

Goldenberries, or dried physalis, which are grown on the foothills of the Andes, are being celebrated as the latest super berry. They are said to contain 166 per cent more antioxidants than cranberries and double the fibre of prunes, and 100 g packs more potassium than four bananas. Still not convinced? They are a rich source of Vitamin C, magnesium, phosphorus and iron. Oh, and with a sharp, sweet flavour, they taste good, too.

ANTIOXIDANTS

Antioxidants are chemicals that occur naturally in fruit, vegetables and other plant foods. They help to repair cell damage in our bodies, preventing a chemical reaction called oxidation, which is caused by free radicals.

Our cells and bodies are constantly being attacked by free radicals in our food, water and air, which can also be created by sun damage, pollution and our own bodies when we are stressed. Free radicals accelerate ageing, destroying collagen, elastin and fibroblasts (the cells responsible for producing these support proteins).

Each type of antioxidant protects our bodies and prevents disease in different ways so it is important to eat as wide a range as possible.

DID YOU KNOW?

A 2012 STUDY AT STANFORD UNIVERSITY IN CALIFORNIA FOUND THAT CHOOSING ORGANIC VEGETABLES REDUCED THE CHANCES OF EATING ANTIBIOTIC-RESISTANT BACTERIA, WHICH ARE THOUGHT TO POSE A SERIOUS RISK TO OUR FUTURE HEALTH.

VITAMIN A

Vitamin A is important for good vision and immune function. It is also essential for skin maintenance and repair; often known as the moisturizing vitamin, it keeps skin smooth, supple and hydrated. There are two forms: retinol, which is found in animal, dairy and fish sources, and beta-carotene, found in fruit, vegetable and plant sources which must be converted in retinol by the body before it can be utilized. It is a fat-soluble vitamin and can be stored by the body.

WARNING Too much retinol can be toxic; it is dangerous for unborn children so pregnant women or those trying to conceive are advised not to follow a high Vitamin A diet. When eaten as beta-carotene in food, it is not dangerous as the body regulates how much is converted into retinol.

GOOD SOURCES OF VITAMIN A INCLUDE

Apricots
Carrots
Dairy products
Egg yolks
Fish
Kale
Liver
Pumpkin
Red peppers
Squash
Sweet potato

VITAMIN C

Vitamin C is essential for collagen production, skin renewal and regrowth and bone formation. It is anti-inflammatory and boosts the immune system, vital for fighting infection, helping blood vessels remain healthy and speeding cell production. It also helps the body to absorb other important vitamins and minerals. As it is water-soluble it cannot be stored by the body and is easily destroyed by cooking or processing.

GOOD SOURCES OF VITAMIN C INCLUDE

Blackcurrants
Citrus fruits
Guava
Kiwi fruit
Leafy green vegetables
Peppers
Radishes
Strawberries
Sweet potato
Tomatoes

HOW
NOT
TO
GET
OLD
202
ANTI-AGEING
FOOD

VITAMIN E

This is one of the most effective antioxidants as it attacks free radicals to protect the skin and prevent tissue and bone damage. Vitamin E maintains healthy muscles, nerves and the reproductive system, helping the body utilize oxygen fully. It also stimulates cell growth and skin healing and reduces inflammation; it even prevents thread and varicose veins. It is best absorbed when eaten with Vitamin C and selenium-rich food. The body's supply needs to be replenished regularly, although it is stored to some degree.

GOOD SOURCES OF VITAMIN E INCLUDE

Almonds and other nuts
Avocados
Fish
Olives
Shellfish
Soya beans
Sunflower seeds
Wheatgerm and oil
Wholegrains

VOLUNTEERS WHO ATE A **WHOPPING SEVENTY ALMONDS A DAY** AS PART OF A CALORIE-CONTROLLED DIET ACTUALLY LOST WEIGHT, A CALIFORNIAN STUDY FOUND. IT'S THOUGHT THAT **THE PROTEIN, FIBRE, EFAS** (ESSENTIAL FATTY ACIDS) AND MONOUNSATURATED FATS IN THE NUTRIENT-RICH NUTS HELPED VOLUNTEERS FEEL SATISFIED AND **LESS PRONE TO CRAVINGS.**

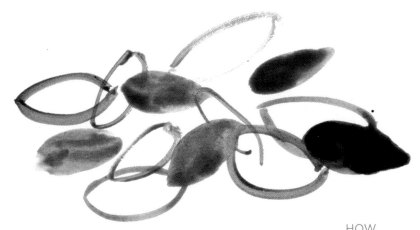

BETA-CAROTENE

This is a carotenoid which forms the red/orange pigment in some root vegetables and fruits; it is also found in some green vegetables where the orange colour is masked by chlorophyll. Carotenoids help to protect against the damaging effects of sunlight.

Beta-carotene is quickly converted into Vitamin A (retinol) in the body where it increases immunity and maintains general health, protecting cell structure and guarding against ageing illnesses. A small amount of fat is necessary to convert it into Vitamin A, so a little olive oil on vegetables helps get the full benefits.

FOODS CONTAINING BETA-CAROTENE INCLUDE

Cantaloupe
Carrots
Collard greens
Coriander (fresh)
Kale
Pumpkin
Spinach
Squash
Sweet potato
Thyme (fresh)
Turnip
Vietnamese gac

LYCOPENE

This is a carotenoid found in tomatoes and other red fruits and vegetables. Lycopene is a powerful antioxidant that works to protect the body from degenerative diseases by helping to neutralize free radicals and prevent DNA damage. High levels of lycopene in the blood and fatty tissues are associated with a reduced risk of cancer, heart disease and macular degeneration. Our bodies do not produce lycopene so it can only be obtained from food sources.

Unlike compounds such as Vitamin C, lycopene is not damaged by cooking. In fact the reverse is true as cooking and processing tomatoes actually increase its strength and usefulness. This makes products such as tomato purée and soup particularly rich sources. Eating tomatoes with oil also helps absorption of lycopene.

FOODS CONTAINING LYCOPENE INCLUDE

Apricots
Goji berries
Papaya
Persimmon
Pink grapefruit
Pink guava
Red peppers
Rosehip
Sea buckthorn
Tomatoes
Vietnamese gac
Watermelon

RESVERATROL

This is a flavonoid found in fruits and in general, the darker the skin of the fruit, the more resveratrol it will contain. It seems to slow DNA ageing in the energy part of cells and protects against inflammation. Flavonoids also boost the body's immune system. Researchers at Harvard Medical School credit the fact that the French have one of the highest ratios of centenarians in the world with their preference for red wine drinking – a good source of resveratrol.

FOODS CONTAINING RESVERATROL INCLUDE
Blackberries
Blackcurrants
Blueberries
Cranberries
Red grapes
Red wine

DID YOU KNOW?

ORGANICALLY GROWN FRUIT AND VEGETABLES REALLY ARE BETTER FOR YOU. RESEARCHERS AT THE UNIVERSITY OF CARDIFF FOUND THAT FRUIT AND VEGETABLES SPRAYED WITH PESTICIDES CONTAIN LOWER LEVELS OF SALICYLATES, THE ACTIVE ANTI-INFLAMMATORY INGREDIENT THAT IS FOUND IN ASPIRIN, AND WHICH HAS BEEN LINKED TO LOWER CANCER RATES.

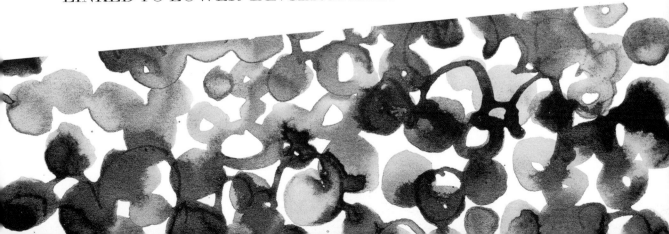

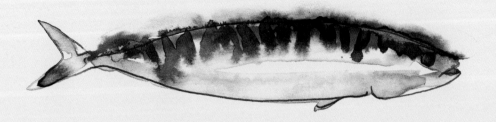

MINERALS

Minerals regulate and balance the body's chemistry. They are needed in only small amounts but are vital for virtually every body process, from boosting the immune system and oxygenating the blood, to controlling blood sugar levels and maintaining healthy skin, bones and teeth. Too much refined, processed food in the diet depletes mineral levels; these need to be replenished in order to stay youthful.

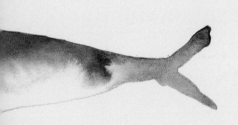

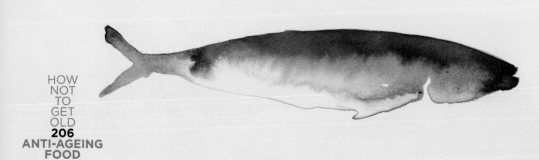

HOW
NOT
TO
GET
OLD
206
**ANTI-AGEING
FOOD**

CALCIUM

Calcium is vital for the formation and maintenance of healthy bones. It guards against osteoporosis as we age. It is also important for healthy skin. To absorb calcium efficiently, your body also needs Vitamin D which is made by your body when it is exposed to sunlight and which is found in oily fish.

GOOD SOURCES OF CALCIUM INCLUDE
Almonds
Dairy products
Oily fish
Tofu
Watercress

SELENIUM

This is a trace element, so your body needs only a small daily amount, but selenium is a powerful antioxidant that protects against premature ageing. It is most effective when combined with Vitamin E.

FOODS CONTAINING SELENIUM INCLUDE
Brazil nuts
Garlic
Mackerel
Sesame seeds
Sunflower seeds

DID YOU KNOW?

EATING JUST FOUR BRAZIL NUTS
WILL GIVE YOU ALL THE SELENIUM
YOUR BODY NEEDS IN A DAY.

HOW
NOT
TO
GET
OLD
207
ANTI-AGEING
FOOD

ZINC

Another trace element, zinc boosts the immune system and energy levels. It is essential for the production of collagen and insulin and it plays an important role in our ability to taste and smell. A lack of zinc shows itself in slow wound healing and dry, damaged hair and nails.

FOODS CONTAINING ZINC INCLUDE

Cheese
Crab
Eggs
Liver
Oysters
Pumpkin seeds
Sardines

SILICA

Silica is essential for the body to create and maintain collagen, making it vital for growth and development. It also has amazing anti-ageing benefits for the skin, helping it to store moisture and thus reducing wrinkles. It's also necessary for shiny, healthy hair and may even slow greying.

FOODS CONTAINING SILICA INCLUDE

Barley
Beetroot
Millet
Oats
Onions
Wholewheat

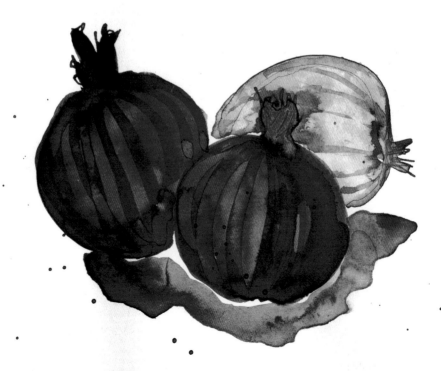

HOW
NOT
TO
GET
OLD
208
**ANTI-AGEING
FOOD**

PROTEIN

Protein is a major component required by our bodies – an essential building block. Everything from muscles, bones, nerves, skin, hair and nails need protein for growth, maintenance and repair. Protein is vital for most bodily processes including metabolism, digestion and the transport of oxygen and nutrients in the blood. It is also necessary for the production of antibodies to fight infection and keeps skin fresh and glowing, bones strong and hair healthy. Proteins release energy slowly into the bloodstream, keeping you alert and quick thinking.

All proteins are built from a combination of twenty-two amino acids and eight of these are essential to our bodies. The amino acids link together to form peptides, or chains. It is the quality of the protein we consume that is important, not the quantity.

GOOD SOURCES OF PROTEIN INCLUDE

Dairy products	Poultry
Eggs	Pulses
Fish	Quinoa
Kidney beans	Shellfish
Meat	Soya beans
Oatmeal	Wholemeal bread

HOW
NOT
TO
GET
OLD
209
**ANTI-AGEING
FOOD**

WONDERFUL WATER

Although not a food, water is absolutely vital for health. Your body is roughly seventy per cent water and you should aim to drink at least two litres every day. And don't rely on feeling thirsty, as the thirst trigger functions less effectively with age.

Water hydrates your skin, smoothing fine lines, flushing out toxins and reducing puffiness. It also improves your circulation and metabolism, helping your body function more effectively.

DID YOU KNOW?

FLUID RETENTION CAN BE MADE WORSE BY DRINKING TOO LITTLE WATER, AS CAN THE APPEARANCE OF CELLULITE.

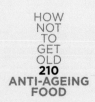

HOW
NOT
TO
GET
OLD
210
**ANTI-AGEING
FOOD**

WHOLE-GRAINS

Wholegrains are the seeds of cereal plants, including oats, wheat, barley, rye and rice. They have a fibre-rich outer layer (the bran) and a nutrient-packed germ. They provide us with B vitamins, folic acid, Omega-3 fatty acids, iron, minerals such as zinc, magnesium and selenium and antioxidant Vitamin E.

Eating more wholegrains can boost the immune system and reduce the risk of heart disease and diabetes, while the fibre they contain encourages healthy digestion.

Breakfast is the ideal opportunity to increase your intake and starting your morning with a satisfying breakfast sets you up for the day. It kick-starts your metabolism and will give you more energy. Skipping breakfast also makes it more likely you'll crave unhealthy snacks later.

Research shows that people who regularly eat breakfast weigh 3.5 kg less on average than those who don't. By choosing healthy wholegrains you'll also lower harmful cholesterol levels.

HOW
NOT
TO
GET
OLD
211
**ANTI-AGEING
FOOD**

THE AGEING ENEMY

Sugar is the enemy of youth. It destroys collagen in your skin and body, and messes with your digestion, resulting in painful bloating, cramps, depression, headaches and lethargy. It also interferes with your blood sugar levels, causing slumps and surges and leading to the storing of sugar as unnecessary fat.

Blood sugar levels can have a damaging effect on skin, causing wrinkles and accelerating the ageing process. High blood sugar triggers a number of chemical reactions, resulting in the creation of free radicals which attack cell membranes. Inflammatory chemicals are then released which cause further damage.

Alongside obviously sugary snacks and drinks, avoid processed foods which often hide vast amounts of sugar. Bear in mind that white carbohydrates including white bread, flour and pasta are quickly turned into glucose, raising sugar levels.

HOW
NOT
TO
GET
OLD
212
ANTI-AGEING
FOOD

RESEARCH FINDINGS

The Human Nutrition Research Centre in Boston set out a series of studies to measure levels of antioxidants in food. Results from the Oxygen Radical Absorbence Capacity, or ORAC, test were used to compile a list of the top-scoring foods. In theory, and it is only a theory, eating more of these could delay the development of wrinkles, improve circulation, memory and brain function, protect joints from arthritis, and even reduce the risk of heart disease and some cancers. It is thought that it is the combination of vitamins, minerals and flavonoids that makes them so effective.

THE TEN TOP-SCORING ORAC FOODS ARE NEARLY ALL HERBS AND SPICES

Dried oregano

Dried rosemary

Dried thyme

Ground cinnamon

Ground cloves

Ground sage

Sorghum bran

Sumac bran

Turmeric

Vanilla beans

HYALURONIC ACID

Hyaluronic acid is the skin's most effective moisturizing agent, effectively working from the inside out. It supports collagen and elastin and researchers claim it can smooth wrinkles.

As we age, the effects of sunlight and free radical damage deplete the amount that is present in skin.

Reports from Yuzuri Hara, a Japanese village two hours from Tokyo where the inhabitants live remarkably long, healthy lives, suggest that the locally grown starchy vegetables are responsible. They are not only a good source of hyaluronic acid, but stimulate the body's own production and are the reason for the villagers' longevity and youthful-looking skin. Good sources of hyaluronic acid are beans, pulses, starchy root vegetables and chicken broth made with bones and skin.

Dr Toyosuke Komori, who works in the village believes that imoji, a potato root and a particular variety of sweet potato are especially beneficial. He commented that he had never seen any cases of skin cancer in the village and it was not unusual for people in their eighties to have spotless skin.

HOW
NOT
TO
GET
OLD
214
**ANTI-AGEING
FOOD**

SIX SIMPLE RULES

FOR ANTI-AGEING NUTRITION

◎ Eat a rainbow of fresh fruits and vegetables, choosing foods from across the colour spectrum to ensure a full-range of anti-ageing nutrients, antioxidants, vitamins and minerals.

◎ Cut down on bad fats and sugars.

◎ Eat more good fats – Omegas 3, 6 and 9 essential fatty acids.

◎ Protein provides the building blocks for healthy, youthful skin, bones and muscles.

◎ Opt for fibre and eat more wholegrains.

◎ Keep well hydrated. Drink plenty of water.

A GUIDE
TO THE
DECADES

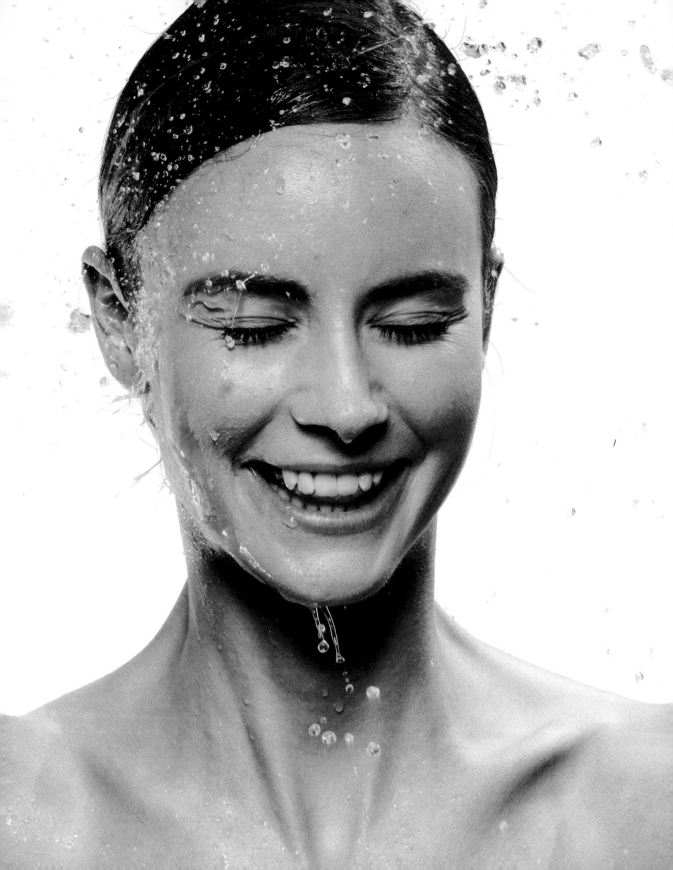

Coco Chanel said, 'Nature gives you the face you have at twenty; it's up to you to merit the face you have at fifty.' For How Not To Get Old's medical expert Doctor Rozina Ali, it's all about taking personal responsibility for the way you look. And you're never too young to start taking care of yourself. What you do in your twenties directly affects the way you age and how young you appear in the following decades.

'People will notice if you look healthy and feel comfortable and confident in yourself', says Rozina. 'Looking good is about how you treat yourself and the world.'

Yes, you can go for a quick fix, but by far the best way to avoid looking old is to build basic care into your everyday routine. Then, later, if you find you need extra help, it can be through subtle maintenance, avoiding the overdone, operated look. 'No one wants to be described as having the kind of face you can buy anywhere', Rozina suggests.

She cites three main culprits when it comes to ageing:

TOP THREE
TO AVOID

SMOKING

Nothing ages you faster. By the time they are thirty, smokers look a good decade older. Pollutants and irritants in smoke break down the skin's support system of collagen and elastin, making it sag and wrinkle. Smoking also starves skin of oxygen and moisture, dulling and drying the complexion.

SUN DAMAGE

Between 85 and 90 per cent of wrinkles are caused by sun damage. Always protect your skin and wear a broad-spectrum sunscreen that guards against UVA and UVB rays.

SUGAR

Research shows the higher the natural levels of blood sugar in your body, the older you look. There's a price to pay for eating refined carbohydrates and sugars which cause glycation of collagen, affecting the speed at which your skin ages.

HOW
NOT
TO
GET
OLD
219
A GUIDE
TO THE
DECADES

YOUR TWENTIES
SIGNS OF AGEING

◎ HORMONES should have settled down, reducing the likelihood of breakouts. Skin will have that youthful glow you'll spend the next decades trying to recapture.

◎ FOR SKIN, the ageing process begins any time between seventeen and twenty-five.

◎ CELL RENEWAL drops by up to 28 per cent by your mid-twenties. After this, the dermis gradually thins; around 1.5 per cent of collagen is lost each year.

◎ BY THE END OF YOUR TWENTIES, your skin is considered mature by cosmetics experts. It will produce less oil and, depending on your lifestyle and genes, the first wrinkles may start appearing.

◎ AT TWENTY, HAIR is at its thickest, although some 20 per cent of men in their twenties experience male pattern baldness. Light-coloured hair can begin to darken. Loss of hair pigment can also become noticeable.

◎ IN TERMS OF THE BODY, any excess fat tends to be distributed fairly evenly. Metabolism and muscle mass will start to decline as body fat increases.

◎ YOUR BONES stop growing around the middle of the decade.

◎ NOW IS THE TIME to set up good habits that will last a lifetime and keep you looking youthful longer.

◎ SOUND SKINCARE is essential. In the morning, cleanse, moisturize and protect your skin from the sun. Wear a cream with at least SPF 15 every day and increase this to a higher factor in summer, or when you're on holiday or likely to be out in the sun. Remember your neck, décolletage and the backs of your hands, which are easy to overlook.

HOW
NOT
TO
GET
OLD
220
**A GUIDE
TO THE
DECADES**

HOW NOT
TO GET OLD

◎ AT NIGHT, get into the habit of cleansing and thoroughly removing any make-up. Dermatologists estimate your skin ages by eight days for every night you sleep in your make-up. Your skin renews and repairs itself while you sleep so it's vital it should be clean and able to breathe. Gentle exfoliants can help to keep skin looking bright and fresh.

◎ CREAMS or treatments containing antioxidants such as Vitamins A, C and E, and minerals including selenium, help to counteract the ageing effects of damaging free radicals in the atmosphere and in the food we eat.

◎ ACNE and similar skin conditions can continue into your twenties. A doctor or skin consultant may prescribe specialist treatment if it's a problem.

◎ IT'S EASY TO THINK you can get away with late nights and early mornings but lack of sleep reduces production of the hormone that controls your body's muscle-to-fat ratio, making it more likely to store fat. It also affects digestion, meaning your body takes 40 per cent longer to regulate blood sugar levels after eating, leaving you with ageing, high sugar levels.

◎ EAT A BALANCED DIET with plenty of fresh fruit and vegetables. It's better for your skin and overall health, and will ultimately influence how well you age. Your bones will continue growing until your mid-twenties, so calcium and omega-3 fatty acids are important. Eating too much sugar, salt and processed foods can lead to a number of health problems later. Yo-yo dieting also overstretches skin, leaving it saggy and wrinkled.

◎ SMOKING ages your heart, lungs and skin, and is a key factor in heart disease and cancer. It can also trigger early menopause and osteoporosis. Just two weeks after giving up you will see an improvement in your skin as circulation recovers to normal levels. Giving up in your twenties will reverse the damage you've done so far.

◎ ALCOHOL is another ageing time bomb. As well as causing bloating and dark circles under your eyes, it dehydrates skin, leading to wrinkles and tired skin that look prematurely old.

◎ EXERCISE is essential to develop lean muscle and strong bones to guard against osteoporosis in later life and boost your metabolic rate now.

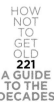

HOW
NOT
TO
GET
OLD
221
**A GUIDE
TO THE
DECADES**

YOUR THIRTIES
SIGNS OF AGEING

◎ CELL RENEWAL slows and skin begins to thin so you lose that youthful bloom.

◎ OIL GLANDS are less active, making skin drier.

◎ AS COLLAGEN AND ELASTIN start to break down, fine lines can develop, particularly frown and nasolabial lines.

◎ FREE RADICAL DAMAGE from smoking, sun and environmental pollution can start to show, with sun spots and areas of uneven pigmentation appearing in your late thirties.

◎ BROKEN VEINS, again as a result of environmental factors, poor diet, alcohol or smoking, can start to appear now as red dots.

◎ ONE IN THREE WOMEN in their thirties use anti-ageing products.

◎ METABOLISM slows by around 0.5 per cent each year. Extra weight tends to settle on the hips for most women and on the abdomen for men.

◎ WITH EACH DECADE, you lose 3.2 kg of lean body mass and there is a slight loss of muscle tone.

◎ FROM THE MID-THIRTIES women start to lose around 1 per cent of bone mass each year.

◎ WOMEN ARE AT THEIR SEXUAL PEAK from their mid-thirties to early forties, though fertility drops around the age of thirty-seven.

◎ TESTOSTERONE production falls in men.

◎ MALE BALDNESS becomes more obvious with thinning hair at the temples and crown.

HOW
NOT
TO
GET
OLD
222
**A GUIDE
TO THE
DECADES**

HOW NOT
TO GET OLD

◎ MAKE SURe your skin creams contain antioxidants and other anti-ageing ingredients. You will probably need a richer moisturizer as skin becomes drier.

◎ IF YOU HAVEN'T ALREADY, start using a specific eye cream for the delicate skin around your eyes which will begin to thin.

◎ BODY BRUSHING before a shower boosts circulation and is good for reducing cellulite.

◎ IF YOU HAVEN'T ALREADY, stop smoking. You can still reverse almost all the damage you've caused.

◎ IT'S EVEN MORE IMPORTANT to eat a healthy, balanced diet rich in the antioxidants you're already using in your face creams, so try to include plenty of foods with the Vitamins A, B, C and E, minerals including selenium, essential oils and supplements like co-enzyme Q10.

◎ VITAMIN A helps to moisturize from the inside so choose foods such as eggs, carrots, sweet potato, peppers, spinach and apricots for naturally plump, hydrated skin.

◎ CUT BACK ON SALT and eat potassium-rich foods including grains, dried fruit, bananas and potatoes to help combat fluid retention and cellulite.

◎ SWAPPING SUGARY, processed foods in favour of complex carbohydrates can help stabilize hormone levels and avoid swings in blood sugar levels.

◎ DRINKING PLENTY OF WATER will keep you hydrated, healthy and looking young, while too much alcohol will encourage the development of red spider veins and pigmentation.

◎ EXERCISE regimes should ideally incorporate some weight-bearing exercise to maintain muscle strength.

◎ REGULAR EXERCISE including brisk walking outdoors helps boost energy levels and mood, as well as maintaining a healthy weight.

◎ LACK OF SLEEP really begins to take a toll now and a good night's rest is vital for your body to repair and rejuvenate.

HOW
NOT
TO
GET
OLD
223
**A GUIDE
TO THE
DECADES**

YOUR FORTIES
SIGNS OF AGEING

◎ AS WOMEN enter the perimenopause, the lead-up to the menopause, oestrogen levels fall, slowing the production of collagen and elastin. It may also bring mood swings, erratic periods, headaches and sometimes depression.

◎ SKIN becomes drier and wrinkles – especially crow's feet, brow and smile lines – become more pronounced.

◎ THE LOSS OF SUBCUTANEOUS FAT leaves skin more fragile and the face looking thinner.

◎ SUDDEN WEIGHT LOSS now will leave baggy, excess skin with no resilience.

◎ SKIN TEXTURE coarsens as dead skin cells build up on the surface.

◎ YOUR JAWLINE begins to lose definition.

◎ AT THE SAME TIME that a woman's face is getting thinner, fat deposits may start to build up on her back and shoulders.

◎ WOMEN'S WAISTS start to thicken and breasts and bottoms begin to sag.

◎ FOR MEN, FAT can build up on the torso but invisible deposits around internal organs can threaten health.

◎ YOUR BODY burns calories more slowly with each decade. It's a sad truth that if you eat the same amount as you did in your twenties, you will put on weight.

◎ HEART AND LUNG capacity reduces by 10–15 per cent.

◎ MEN AND WOMEN in their forties will start to notice a loss of flexibility and muscle strength.

◎ GREY HAIRS become much more obvious for men and women, and baldness accelerates for men.

◎ MEN also experience increased irritability and tiredness.

◎ VISION declines.

HOW NOT TO GET OLD

◎ SKIN PROTECTION - against sun and environmental damage – is even more important.

◎ SKIN WILL BE DRIER so switch to a richer moisturizer with antioxidants to counteract free radical damage.

◎ EXFOLIATION and moisturizing skin facials will help to improve texture and keep skin looking younger.

◎ STRESS AND LACK OF SLEEP are often the side effects of a hectic lifestyle, balancing the needs of family, work and home. Your body will cope less well and the higher levels of adrenaline and the stress hormone cortisol play havoc with skin, blood sugar and your immune system. Try to take time out for yourself to relax and recharge.

◎ REGULAR EXERCISE will counteract muscle and skeletal wastage, keep you toned and boost your metabolism.

◎ CHOOSE WEIGHT-BEARING EXERCISE and anything that encourages flexibility such as Pilates or yoga. Avoid high-impact exercise such as jogging, which can exacerbate facial sagging and joint weakness.

◎ THINK ABOUT YOUR DIET. What you ate in your thirties may no longer fit your body's needs. Hormone- and oestrogen-balancing foods will help you avoid feeling and looking your age.

◎ EAT FAT - not all fats are bad. Essential fatty acids found in oily fish, nuts and seeds are antioxidant, anti-inflammatory, good for your overall health and great for your skin, leaving it smoother and better hydrated.

HOW
NOT
TO
GET
OLD
225
**A GUIDE
TO THE
DECADES**

YOUR FIFTIES
SIGNS OF AGEING

◎ SKIN IS THINNER, DRIER and more fragile. Rough patches and open pores from past sun damage become more noticeable.

◎ YOUR COMPLEXION is increasingly sallow with no youthful blush.

◎ LINES DEEPEN into folds and the loss of tissue and slow renewal of collagen increases facial sagging, especially cheeks and jowls.

◎ OESTROGEN LEVELS really drop with the onset of the menopause. Half of all women experience hot flushes, night sweats, joint pain, memory loss and headaches.

◎ THERE IS ALSO A RISK of osteoporosis as bones thin.

◎ YOUR BODY BURNS FEWER calories and stores more fat which tends to head for the waist, thighs, buttocks, abdomen, chin and even under the eyes – basically everywhere you don't want it.

◎ FOR MEN, weight continues to accumulate on the abdomen and there will be a greater risk of cardiovascular and circulatory disease.

◎ STAMINA, ENERGY and bone mass decline.

◎ LIBIDO DROPS for both sexes.

◎ VISION gets worse.

◎ GREY HAIRS MULTIPLY (on the body, too), but overall, men will have less hair.

◎ NAILS thicken and can develop ridges.

HOW
NOT
TO
GET
OLD
226
**A GUIDE
TO THE
DECADES**

HOW NOT TO GET OLD

◎ RICH ANTI-AGEING SKIN CREAMS can help moisturize and restore skin's balance.

◎ CHOOSE GENTLE EXFOLIANTS and peels to strip away dead skin cells and stimulate collagen production.

◎ DIET can really help ease the symptoms of the menopause. Vitamins, minerals and essential fatty acids are vital. A nutritionist can advise on a specific eating plan and supplements. Eating wholegrains and plenty of fibre can help balance hormones.

◎ EXERCISE continues to be important if you want to maintain bone density and muscle mass.

◎ IF YOU STOP SMOKING at fifty it will still make a positive difference to your health and appearance, effectively turning your body clock back six years.

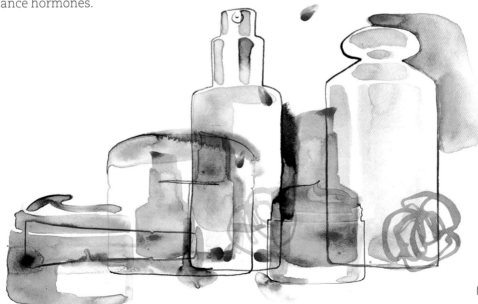

HOW
NOT
TO
GET
OLD
227
**A GUIDE
TO THE
DECADES**

YOUR SIXTIES
SIGNS OF AGEING

◎ SKIN generally loses pigment. The pigment cells, or melamolytes, that you are left with tend to clump together to form sun or age spots.

◎ DEEPER FACIAL LINES develop and the neck shows greater wrinkling and sagging.

◎ UNDEREYE BAGS develop.

◎ SKIN is noticeably thinner and increasingly less elastic.

◎ THE SKIN'S RATE OF RENEWAL and repair slows down.

◎ WOMEN MAY NOTICE an increase in facial hair as a result of the drop in oestrogen and a rise in testosterone levels post menopause.

◎ THE DROP IN OESTROGEN levels triggers body changes, with more weight on the hips and often increased breast size.

◎ METABOLIC RATES FALL. The average seventy-year-old burns five hundred fewer calories each day than a twenty-five-year-old.

◎ THE NOSE AND EARLOBES lengthen and men may notice an increase in hair growth in these areas.

◎ MALE BALDING accelerates while there will be a reduction in body hair.

◎ THERE IS FURTHER MUSCLE wastage and an increased risk of osteoporosis for women.

◎ THE RISK OF CARDIOVASCULAR disease increases for both men and women.

◎ MANY PEOPLE notice a decline in their short-term memory.

HOW
NOT
TO
GET
OLD
228
**A GUIDE
TO THE
DECADES**

HOW NOT
TO GET OLD

◎ CONTINUE using rich anti-ageing products and sun protection to nourish and even skin tone.

◎ FACIAL MASSAGE and exercise can help to stimulate deep tissue and improve circulation.

◎ YOGA AND PILATES are good weight-bearing forms of exercise to maintain bone and muscle strength. Swimming can help ease stiff joints and muscles.

◎ OMEGA-3 and other essential fatty acids help keep your brain working – they are also wonderful for skin.

◎ THE NEED FOR B VITAMINS increases with age. They are vital for a healthy cardiovascular system and can help avoid memory loss.

◎ ZINC, found in shellfish, wholegrains, beans and peas, also helps concentration and memory.

◎ THE BODY PRODUCES less Vitamin D – essential for the absorption of calcium and maintenance of healthy bones and skin. Our bodies make Vitamin D through exposure to sunlight and it is also found in oily fish and fish oils. However, the British Nutrition Foundation recommends everyone over sixty-five should take a Vitamin D supplement.

HOW
NOT
TO
GET
OLD
229
**A GUIDE
TO THE
DECADES**

AGE-APPROPRIATE PROCEDURES

There's growing evidence that far from keeping you looking youthful, having too much done too young can actually be ageing and in some cases damaging. *How Not To Get Old* asked Dr Rozina Ali which procedures may be appropriate in different decades. These are her suggestions:

IN YOUR TWENTIES

◎ FOR MOST PEOPLE IN THEIR TWENTIES, no major anti-ageing treatments will be necessary. Facials and massage can all boost your sense of well-being, brightening dull complexions and kick starting sluggish circulation.

◎ IF YOU HAVE A MAJOR ISSUE with your appearance or something that you've always wanted to change, such as ear correction or nose reshaping, now is probably a good time to consider it as you can benefit from it for the rest of your life.

◎ MEN WHO ARE GENETICALLY PREDISPOSED to male pattern baldness may consider a hair transplant.

HOW
NOT
TO
GET
OLD
230
**A GUIDE
TO THE
DECADES**

IN YOUR THIRTIES

◎ YOU COULD START THINKING about using Botox® on lines.

◎ FILLERS SUCH AS HYALURONIC ACID (HA) fillers, calcium hydroxylapatite and Sculptra® can all help to combat the loss of youthful plumpness.

◎ EXFOLIATION THROUGH GENTLE SKIN PEELS can brighten and revitalize dull complexions.

IN YOUR FORTIES

◎ GENTLE RADIOFREQUENCY SKIN TIGHTENING such as Pellevé and IPL can help combat sagging on face and body.

◎ FEEL-GOOD TREATMENTS including mesotherapy help rejuvenate complexions, bringing a youthful glow.

◎ NON-SURGICAL PROCEDURES are still the most appropriate for your face at this point.

◎ BOTOX® TREATMENTS - perhaps just twice a year – can reduce wrinkles while fillers can plump and contour hollow temples and cheeks, and thinning lips.

◎ TRETINOIN used at night can have an anti-ageing effect but this is a prescription-only cream and there can be side effects, notably skin drying or redness, and you will need a liver function test first. It should also never be used if you are, or are trying to become, pregnant.

◎ A BREAST LIFT can reshape as well as raise, restoring a pre-breastfeeding appearance.

HOW
NOT
TO
GET
OLD
231
**A GUIDE
TO THE
DECADES**

IN YOUR FIFTIES

◎ FILLERS can plump up lips and cheeks.

◎ LOSS OF ELASTICITY, crepiness, and expression lines around eyes can result in drooping eyelids or undereye bags – these could be solved by blepharoplasty (eyelid surgery).

◎ RADIOFREQUENCY SKIN TIGHTENING TECHNIQUES such as Thermage can smooth and contour ageing skin on the body, including arms and stomach, as well as the face.

◎ LASERS OR SCLEROTHERAPY can treat red spider veins on legs or other parts of the body.

◎ ABDOMINOPLASTY, OR A TUMMY TUCK, can remove excess skin and fat on the stomach and waist following pregnancies or major weight loss.

IN YOUR SIXTIES

◎ SKIN REJUVENATION using IPL or lasers can help combat sun damage.

◎ FACE OR NECK LIFTS at this stage can turn back the clock to reverse some of the most obvious signs of ageing.

◎ UPPER OR LOWER EYELID SURGERY removes excess skin and can make eyes appear more open and youthful.

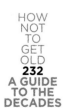
HOW
NOT
TO
GET
OLD
232
**A GUIDE
TO THE
DECADES**

DIRECTORY

ACUPUNCTURE
British Acupuncture Council
63 Jeddo Road, London W12 9HQ
Tel: 020 8735 0400
www.acupuncture.org.uk

AROMATHERAPY
**International Federation of
Professional Aromatherapists**
Tel: 01455 637987
www.ifparoma.org

COSMETIC AND PLASTIC SURGERY
**The British Association of
Aesthetic Plastic Surgeons
The Royal College of Surgeons of England**
35–43 Lincoln's Inn Fields, London WC2A 3PE
Tel: 020 7430 1840
www.baaps.org.uk

**The British Association
of Plastic Surgery**
www.baps.co.uk

**The British Association of Plastic,
Reconstructive and Aesthetic Surgeons**
The Royal College of Surgeons
35–43 Lincoln's Inn Fields
London WC2A 3PE
Tel: 020 7831 5161
www.bapras.org.uk

**International Society of
Aesthetic Plastic Surgery**
www.isaps.org

The General Medical Council
Regent's Place, 350 Euston Road
London NW1 3JN
www.gmc-uk.org

**The Cosmetic Imaging Studio
(Nick Miedzianowski-Sinclair)**
Queen Anne Street Medical Centre
18–20 Queen Anne Street
London W1G 8HU
TEL: 0777 802409
www.thecosmeticimagingstudio.com

Dr Rozina Ali
**Consultant Plastic and
Reconstructive Surgeon**
Email: rsa.plasticsurgery@gmail.com
www.rozinaali.com

Mr Stephen Hamilton
**Consultant Plastic, Reconstructive
and Cosmetic Surgeon**
Tel: 020 7432 8266
Email: info@stephenhamilton.org.uk
www.stephenhamilton.org.uk

Mr Christopher Inglefield
**Plastic, Reconstructive and
Cosmetic Surgeon
London Bridge Plastic Surgery**
54 Wimpole Street, London W1G 8YG
Tel: 020 7487 0900
www.lbps.co.uk

Mr Barry M. Jones
**Consultant Plastic and
Reconstructive Surgeon**
14a Upper Wimpole Street
London W1G 6LR
Tel: 020 7935 1938
www.barrymjones.co.uk

Mr Alex Karidis
Plastic and Cosmetic Surgeon
3rd Floor, 60 Grove End Road
London NW8 9NH
Tel: 020 7432 8727
www.nipntuck.co.uk

HOW
NOT
TO
GET
OLD
233
DIRECTORY

Mr Adrian Richards
10 Harley Street, London W1G 9PF
Tel: 0800 652 5902
www.adrianrichards.com

Mr Taimur Shoaib
Consultant Plastic Surgeon
www.shoaib.co.uk

NON-SURGICAL COSMETIC PRACTITIONERS
The British Association of Dermatologists
Willan House, 4 Fitzroy Square
London W1T 5HQ
Tel: 020 7383 0266
www.bad.org.uk

Dr Sam Bunting
Cosmetic Dermatologist
10 Harley Street, London W1G 9PF
Tel: 020 7467 8493
www.drsambunting.com

Sarah Chapman
Skincare expert and founder
of Skinesis Clinic
106 Draycott Avenue, London SW3 3AE
Tel: 020 7589 9585
www.sarahchapman.net

Dr Vicky Dondos
Cosmetic Doctor
Medicetics
Tel: 020 3051 2816
www.medicetics.com

Dr Maurice Dray
Cosmetic doctor, dermatologist
and gerontologist
11b Albert Place, London W8 5PD
Tel: 020 7937 1031
www.drdray.co.uk

Dr Tracy Mountford
Founder and Medical Director
of The Cosmetic Skin Clinic
10 Harley Street, London W1G 9PF
or
84 Rogers Lane, Stoke Poges
Buckinghamshire SL2 4LF
Tel: 01753 646660
www.cosmeticskinclinic.com

Dr Tapan Patel
Founder and Medical Director
of VIVA Clinic
Golders Hill Houe
592 Finchley Road
London NW11 7RX
Tel: 020 8455 4460
www.viva-clinic.co.uk

Dr Rita Rakus
Cosmetic Doctor
34 Hans Road, London SW3 1RW
Tel: 020 7460 7324
www.drrritarakus.com

Dr Daniel Sister
Cosmetic and Aesthetic
Medical Practitioner
8–9 Lambton Place
London W11 2SH
Tel: 020 7221 2248
www.drdanielsister.com

Dr Maryam Zamani
Opthalmologist and
Aesthetic Practitioner
120 Sloane Street
London SW1X 9BW
Tel: 0870 864 8500
www.drmaryamzamani.com

COSMETIC DENTISTRY
British Academy of Cosmetic Dentistry
29 Harley Street, London W1G 9QR
Tel: 020 7612 4166
www.bacd.com

British Dental Association
64 Wimpole Street, London W1G 8YS
Tel: 020 7935 0875
www.bda.org

Dr Charles Adam E. Slade
United Smile Centres
Lister House, 11–12 Wimpole Street
London W1G 9ST
Tel: 0800 849 4959
www.unitedsmilecentres.co.uk

EXERCISE
Boxercise
Tel: 0844 7705 333
www.boxercise.co.uk

European Health and Fitness Association
www.ehfa.eu.com

Hula Hooping
Hooper Street
Email: hooperstreete1@gmail.com
www.hooperstreet.co.uk

National Register of Personal Trainers
www.nrpt.co.uk

Walking Workouts
Email: info@walkingworkouts.co.uk
www.walkingworkouts.co.uk

HAIR
Mr Edward Ball
Tel: 07769 683326
www.doctoredwardball.com

The Hospital Group
Tel: 08457 626 727
www.thehospitalgroup.org

Ziering Medical
Tel: 0808 149 7281
www.hairtransplantziering.co.uk

MAKE-UP
Wild about Beauty
Email: info@wildaboutbeauty.com
www.wildaboutbeauty.com

NUTRITION
Elizabeth Peyton-Jones
Author of *Eat Yourself Young*
Email: info@epjhealth.com
www.epjhealth.com

PILATES
The Pilates Foundation
PO Box 51186
London SE13 9DA
Tel: 020 7033 0078
www.pilatesfoundation.com

REFLEXOLOGY
Association of Reflexologists
5 Fore Street, Taunton
Somerset TA1 1HX
Tel: 01823 351010
www.aor.org.uk

YOGA
Danielle Collins
The Danielle Collins Face Yoga Method
www.faceyogaexpert.com

Yoga Workshops and Yoga Teacher Training
Tel: 020 7042 9900/01
www.yogacampus.com

Yoga Biomedical Trust
Email: enquiries@yogatherapy.org
www.yogatherapy.org

HOW
NOT
TO
GET
OLD
235
DIRECTORY

INDEX

HOW
NOT
TO
GET
OLD
236
INDEX

HOW
NOT
TO
GET
OLD
238
INDEX

ACKNOWLEDGEMENTS

I would like to thank all those who shared their stories or contributed their valuable expert knowledge. Special thanks to: Dr Rozina Ali, Louise Redknapp, Max Pemberton, Anna Richardson, Dr Tracy Mountford and Jean Beard at The Cosmetic Skin Clinic, Victoria Kidd at The Hospital Group, Elizabeth Peyton-Jones, Danielle Collins, Gill Wilson, Tim Carter, Lisa Edwards, Kirsty Hanson, Jen Fazey, Viv Pheysey, Ana de Moraes, Hana Canter, Sarah Fink and the Twenty Twenty production and research teams, Michelle Signore and all at Transworld Publishers, Clare Sayer and Smith & Gilmour for their design.

HOW
NOT
TO
GET
OLD
239
INDEX

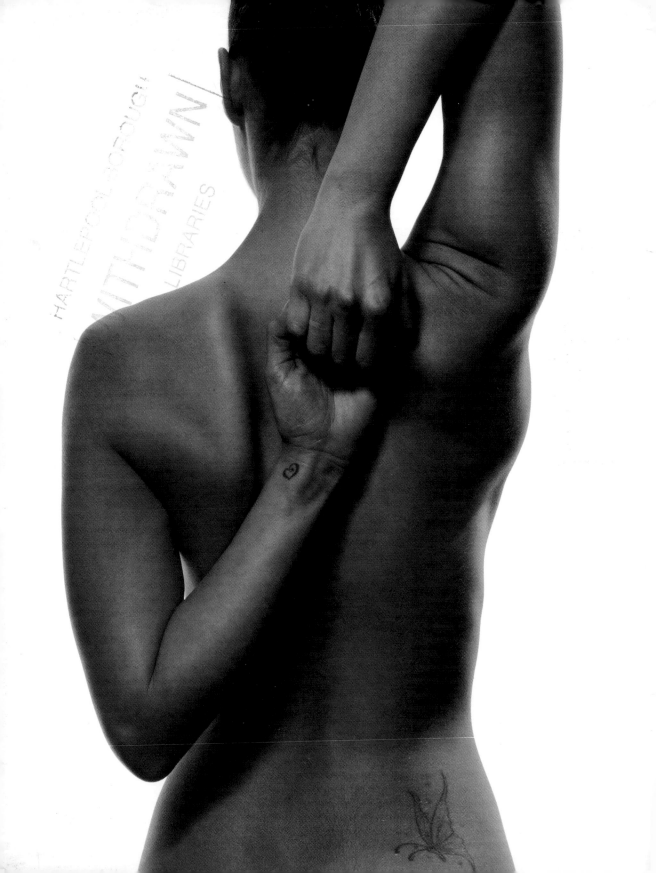